ACHIEVING WELLNESS THROUGH RISK TAKING

To my parents, who let me climb to the far reaches of our backyard cherry tree when I was but a toddler, knowing that I might fall. And fall I did, even broke an arm, though I thank them for those experiences because I learned that there are limbs in life which, like the cherry tree, break if you don't climb with caution, experimenting as you go.

I thank them for their constant patience, for always having time to answer the many questions prompted by my immense curiosity, for letting me explore my world and letting me conquer the dining room table and, finally, that cherry tree. For in all things worthwhile there is a risk. But cherries on higher limbs swell larger with sweetness because they catch more sun; so I discovered the risk of climbing higher was always worth the sweeter taste of mastery.

So, to my parents, who let me challenge my small world; who let me fail, yet were always there to say, "You can do it, honey," I dedicate this book.

ACHIEVING
WELLNESS
THROUGH
RISK TAKING

THE END OF BOREDOM

by

Dr. Mark Crookse

Exposition Press of Florida, Inc.   Pompano Beach, Florida

FIRST EDITION

©1985 by Dr. Mark Crookse

Library of Congress Catalog Card Number: 85-90954

ISBN 0-682-40249-4

Printed in the United States of America

Contents

Acknowledgements

The author wishes to acknowledge the following people who made significant contributions to this effort;

Dr. Don Ardell for his periodic review of the manuscript and his well-timed suggestions. Don also helped germinate the concept of heroic acts as a form of spiritual uplifting in his own book *14 Days To Wellness* even as I was formulating the same general belief. Don's Wellness Continuum was slightly changed to represent the role boredom plays in our efforts to reach a high state of mental and physical well-being.

Dr. Hal Becker, for coming all the way to Kansas City to monitor my psychological state during the sensory deprivation tests and for his use of Sub-Liminal Communication, which helped immeasurably.

Dr. Donald Vest at Washburn University, who assisted in large degree in the writing of Chapter 9 and who was always there to spur me on in my sensation-seeking lifestyle. Don provided much insights and reading material on the subject of risk taking.

Dr. Norge Jerome, Dr. Richard Harris, and Dr. Charles Rudolph for their assistance in the nutrition chapter and for their ideas and suggestions on optimal nutrition.

Preface

Human beings cannot survive alone on air, water, food, and shelter. Like all other animals, we need sensory stimulation in order to prevent boredom. As my research has taught me, some of us have greater requirements than others. We will go to great lengths to fulfill this biologically determined need, even when the risks are great. It's kind of like the moth in Don Marquis's little poem:

The Lesson Of The Moth

Fire is beautiful
and we know that
if we get too close it will kill us
but what does that matter?
it is better to be happy for a moment
and be burned up in beauty
than to be bored all the while
and so the little moth
went and immolated himself
on a patent cigar lighter

Like the moth, we also crave excitement. The flame for us is our highly structured and regimented twentieth-century world. Our nervous systems were never designed for monotony, but rather for variation and novelty. So, it's easy to become bored in a world where the environment is under such extensive control.

If we can take a backward glance (which we will frequently do in this book), we may begin to understand that,

Primitive man had a much greater sense of himself than we do today . . . he was in touch with his inner processes. . . . He regarded as inseparable his body, mind, and spirit.

Our ancestors were high risk takers. Survival demanded it. But the once-natural forms of risk taking have been drastically altered in our race forward.

The supermarket aisle has replaced the hunt, the automobile has replaced exploration by foot, and the secondhand has replaced the movement of a shadow across the Earth.

Boredom is a powerful force that molds much of human behavior. Unwilling to steep myself in alcohol, to get "high" on substances that can dull even the finest minds, or to engage in some other abberant social behaviors that characterize our times, I chose to engage myself in some dangerous stunts in order to deal with a lifestyle which was, for all intents and purposes, as predictable as the law of gravity. But with my adventures came a philosophy based upon control of life's uncertain events. As the Garden of Eden story shows, we have free will. We can help shape our destinies much more than most of us care to admit. That's why in this book I have chosen to view much of human behavior through the binoculars of the risk taker, for in every human action there is gain or loss involved.

Please do not ever attempt any of these stunts or feats. They were specific to my life and times. There are many other challenges to serve your own growth. Enjoy them for what they were; the catalyst that led me to the writing of this book and the lessons herein contained.

Introduction

We are all risk takers; there is no way to avoid taking risks. Such behaviors, whether purposeful or by habit, are part of our everyday lives, though most of us fail to recognize this fact.

You took a risk when you got up this morning. But think of this; maybe staying in bed was a risk with more undesirable consequences, even though it had some short-term attractions.

You took another risk when you bought this book. So did the bookseller who stocked it, the publisher who printed it, and especially the man who wrote it.

The author, a remarkable athlete with the insatiable curiosity all great scientists must have, probably takes fewer negative risks than you, or the average person for that matter. Yet he takes *many* risks, because he goes in search of wellness. He takes positive risks that have value in terms of personal growth and knowledge—and he had the energy and creativity to develop a system from his own experiments that can have great implications for your future well-being and happiness.

From 1980 to 1982 I studied positive risk takers. I gathered data, conducted interviews, mailed questionnaires, and read articles and testimonials about people who performed "heroic deeds" of endurance and mental toughness. I wanted to know how these prodigious pursuits, all of which were divorced from necessity or survival, affected the risk taker's experience of self-responsibility, nutritional patterns, overall fitness levels, ability to manage and direct stress energies, and sense of psychological/spiritual/cultural well-being.

What I discovered was a strong association between "heroic acts" and wellness lifestyles, as long as certain principles guided the heroic quest. I hinted at some of these qualities but left most of the potent questions for someone else. "Someone else" wrote this book. He based his analysis not only on a study of others but on his own experiential learning through a succession of impressive heroic acts.

Mark Crookse has discovered the ultimate antidote to the worseness of low-level boredom–high-level risk taking for wellness. And he did it the old-fashioned way; he earned it.

You are in for a treat. *Achieving Wellness Through Risk Taking: The End of Boredom* is at once a tale of adventure, a text on the principles and approaches to optimal health, and an inspirational pep talk. When you finish, it is unlikely you will settle for anything less than being the best you can.

DONALD B. ARDELL, PH.D.

SECTION I

Introduction: Wellness and Risk Taking

Boredom is a product of modern society. Primitive people rarely suffered from boredom. Each day was a lesson in survival, meeting the demands of the environment or exploring new opportunities. They measured time by the shadow; they lived in harmony with nature.

The opposite of boredom is enthusiasm, the feeling of excitement and eager anticipation at life's possibilities. We all can experience enthusiasm frequently if we apply the wellness concepts, as I'll show. *The end of boredom is near.* What about that weird-sounding word, *wellness?* What is it?

Wellness means optimal, rather than "normal," health, giving up any notions you have that getting by or coping is all there is. It's achieved by implementing the seven components shown in the illustration on page 2.

Like the wheel's strength the quality and quantity of our lives, are determined by how well we utilize these seven components, Briefly, they are:

1. *Uniqueness.* Establishing your unique identity, daring to discover those unusual talents and traits that differentiate you from others. What a dull, boring world it would be if we were all "designed with uniformity in mind."
2. *Stress Management.* Learning to relax and let go of tensions. Skills such as knowing how to communicate or visualize can turn stress into a positive force so peak performances can be reached.
3. *Sensitivity.* Compassion for others, loving and sharing with those less fortunate. Creating optimal surroundings at home or work to promote satisfaction. This component is a calling to our spiritual selves.
4. *Safety.* Managing the physical environment at home, at work, in travel, and in sports to minimize any potential health hazards.
5. *Nutrition.* Gaining awareness of our food intake. Why do I eat what

1

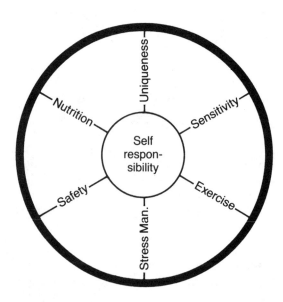

The Wellness Model ● With any of the components missing, the strength of the wheel is weakened, and the risk of breaking increases.

> I do and how can nutrition help me be a healthier, more energetic person?
>
> 6. *Exercise*. Being fit for life, for work, for play. Regaining the Greek ideal of balance, a strong mind in a strong body. Discovering new limits.
> 7. *Self-responsibility*. Assuming control of the above components that determine our health. This is *risk taking*, weighing the pros and cons of our thoughts, behaviors, and actions. This is the most important part, the key to self-improvement.

All this simply means setting challenges, leaving the world of mediocrity. If you settle for mediocrity, eventually you'll become bored, like so many other "normal" people. As the wellness continuum (illustrated on page 3) shows, this often leads to poor risk behaviors which leads to disease. "Death by Boredom" isn't just a euphemism. It is an everyday reality, a reality born of life in highly urbanized environments. So, you'll have to risk.

The greater your challenge, the greater will be your risks. Still, by utilizing wellness principles, you learn to identify situations, people, foods, and behaviors that endanger your success. (Such potential dangers are called *risk factors*). Positive risk takers throw loaded dice in the "Monop-

The Wellness Continuum

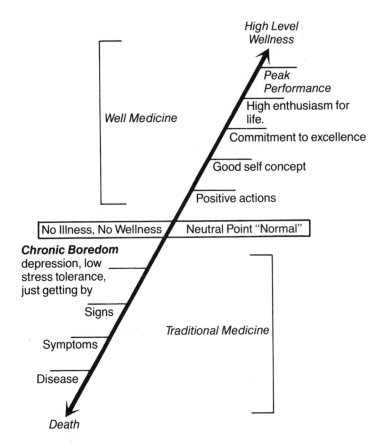

oly Game" of life. By managing risks, their successes far outnumber their mistakes.

Our potent need for stimulation clouds much of our decision making and our instincts no longer guide us. We need to regain the balance we lost to Madison Avenue's brand of happiness

In this section, I'll discuss the problem of boredom, test you in the seven components of wellness in the Life Risk Questionnaire, and describe my own odyssey to escape boredom. The remainder of the book will focus on each of these seven wellness areas.

CHAPTER 1

Boredom and Risk Taking

Could it be that the middle-class life of prosperity, while satisfying our material needs leaves us with a feeling of intense boredom, and that suicide and alcoholism are pathological ways of escaping from this boredom? Could it be that [the high incidence of both these behaviors in the United States] is a drastic illustration of the truth that . . . modern civilization fails to satisfy profound needs in man? If so, what are these needs?

—Erich Fromm, *The Sane Society*

Chronic Boredom—Origins and Health Implications

Are you bored? If so, join the crowd. Millions of Americans wrestle with boredom day after day, many not fully understanding the origin or the way out of this dilemma. In our society chronic boredom is not considered a behavioral disorder, or a sickness, or even a state of maladjustment, it is so pervasive (normal) an occurrence. The word boredom cannot be found in the index of any abnormal psychology text. And yet, a search of the scientific literature firmly establishes its relationship to crime and drug abuse in teenagers, to the frequency of injury and illness in industry, and even to the incidence of heart disease.

Usually, those who suffer the most are blue-collar workers whose jobs offer little or no opportunity for growth, advancement, or for that matter *any change at all* from the monotonous, regimented, routine of the workplace. Consider the following quote from Kanter and Stein's *Life In Organizations*.

The assembly line carries 101 cars past each worker every hour. A worker has thirty-six seconds to perform his assigned snaps, knocks, or squirts on each car . . . The job had been boring before, but [after more snaps, knocks, or squirts were required], there was a 97% vote to strike . . . "It's not the money, it pays good, but it's driving me crazy." It's the job everyone said,

4

but they found it hard to describe . . . what's there to say? A car comes, I weld it. A car comes, I weld it. A car comes, I weld it. 101 times an hour.

I asked a young wife, "What does your husband tell you about your work?" "He doesn't say what he does. Only if something happened like, 'My hair caught on fire', or 'Something fell in my face'".

"There's a lot of variety in the paint shop", said a dapper twenty-two year old. You clip on the color hose, bleed out the old color, and squirt. Clip, bleed, squirt, yawn; clip, bleed, squirt, scratch your nose. Only now there's no time to scratch your nose."

"How do you keep from going crazy?" I asked.

"I have fantasies. You know what I keep imagining? I see a car coming down. It's red, so I know it's gonna have a black seat, black dash, black interiors. But I keep thinking what if somebody up there sends down the wrong color interiors—like orange, and me putting in yellow cushions, bright yellow!

"There's always water fights, paint fights, or laugh, talk, tell jokes, anything so you don't feel like a machine . . . you're always waiting for the line to break down."

It is no wonder that such people often take to alcohol in excessive quantities, smoke more and more cigarettes, overconsume foods, and engage in deviant sexual behaviors in order to cope.

Until after the Jefferson era ours was an agricultural society. When everyone was fairly well accountable for his or her own survival it bestowed a feeling that, good times or bad, one had some degree of control over life. But the major technological advances soon brought a halt to that: the spinning jenny, the cotton gin, the first Model-T that rolled off the assembly line in 1913, the first flight at Kitty Hawk, all were part of the quantum leap that ushered in mass production, job specialization, and boredom as never before.

But there was nothing inherently wrong with such advances, because it is a truism of human nature that we have a need to progress, to improve the state of things. The problem was that somewhere in this frenzied rush we forgot that people are more than producers of products and services, that they feel, think, create, and desire growth. To deny access to such expressions is to create a machine, a machine of the very worst kind, a machine that will break down in the final analysis, affecting all of us. Education creates more opportunity, true, but worker satisfaction still hinges on two things: continued challenge and avoiding a monotonous routine of high predictability.

In 1973, the U.S. Department of Health, Education, and Welfare issued, *Work in America*, a report that captured the attention of the public as few government reports do. The report focused on the alienation in the American work force, and because of it "blue collar blues" and "white collar woes" were suddenly recognized as a serious problem in American economic life. It stated:

> Significant numbers of American workers are dissatisfied with the quality of their working lives. Dull, repetitive, seemingly meaningless tasks, offering little challenge or autonomy, are causing discontent among workers at all occupational levels.

The University of Michigan's Institute for Social Reform, which conducted national surveys of worker satisfaction in 1969, 1973, and 1977, showed a continued rise in job dissatisfaction—especially among college graduates.

Work In America reported that, when asked if they would choose the same jobs over again, 57 percent of the college graduates and 76 percent of the blue-collar workers said no. This report also found that worker satisfaction was a better predictor of life expectancy than the traditional diagnostic measures uncovered during a medical exam, like high blood pressure, smoking history, etc.

A similar study on females found that satisfaction with life situations was more closely correlated with health than were the occupations per se. It mattered not whether a woman was "just a housewife" or was employed in some business; the single most important factor in predicting health was boredom. Perhaps this is the greatest source of distress people face today.

All of us need excitement with appropriate stimulation. We need it just as certainly as we need air, food, water, and shelter. The search for food is not too exciting today, it is (as so many things are today) very predictable. Stimulation seeking comes in many forms. It involves decision making—risk taking if you will—aimed at satisfying this powerful need. Unfortunately, rapid urbanization and technological advances tend to deny us the more natural forms of risk-taking behaviors. As Desmond Morris, writing in *The Human Zoo,* explains,

> There are solutions. One is a rather drastic one. It is a variation of the stimulus struggle called tempting survival. The disillusioned teenager, instead of throwing a ball on a playing field, can throw it through a plate glass window. The disillusioned housewife, instead of stroking the dog can stroke the milkman. The disillusioned businessman, instead of stripping down the engine of his car can strip down his secretary. In no time at all the individual is involved in the true survival struggle of fighting for his life.

To combat boredom, people may resort to extremes of behavior which border on savagery. Medical annals tell of an older female, unable to knit because of arthritis, who progressed from nail biting, to skin chewing, to bone gnawing until the terminal bone of her middle finger had been chewed away. Proper prescribed stimulation halted the behavior.

We have, it seems, become confused. We take the wrong kinds of risks. The more natural forms of risk-taking behaviors (hunting, defending territory, or problem solving in the environment) were part of our heritage. For eons they fulfilled our needs for stimulation. As a species, we cannot slough off the impact of our 2-million-year history in eighty short years. So, the comforts and securities of the twentieth century lure us into a sense of complacency and we look to artificial forms of sensation and risk taking to satisfy these needs.

This book will help you better understand the entire concept of risk taking and to avoid some of the entrapments that wind up causing distress, discontentment, and even despair. The pursuit of high-level wellness is the aim of this book, reaching your full potential, and thus experiencing more life satisfaction.

If Thoreau's Walden Pond was the first "Wellness Retreat" from the quiet desperation of our times, then Madison Avenue is the Olympics of herd conformity and social pathology.

In a society where tuning up the car is more important than tuning up the body, where a "Great Idea" is dissected by a committee and put in the freezer because "parts is parts," where bikini-clad women have orgasms on television spreading Erotica Shaving Cream all over Superbowl Joe's crusty face, where Marlboro Cowboys watch sunsets disappear on the horizon through a mist of cigarette smoke, it's no wonder we wind up confused and feeling lost. Wellness through risk taking will help you find the way out.

The first step is to have you begin by taking the Life Risk Questionnaire in this chapter to find where you are at present in terms of risk-taking behaviors. Be as honest as you can. This is for you alone; it will serve as a guide to highlight areas which need work as you read through this book.

Life Risk Questionnaire

Social-Emotional Risks	Often	Sometimes	Rarely
1. Do you experience depression?	5	3	0
2. Do you feel life is helpless and you have no control over your life events?	5	3	0
3. Do you hold your emotions in (fail to express anger, criticism, emotional needs)?	5	3	0
4. Do you feel in conflict with others, are you feeling distressed?	5	3	0
5. Are you suicidal?	5	3	0

Social-Emotional Risks	Often	Sometimes	Rarely
6. Do you feel lonely?	2	1	0
7. Do you get deeply involved with someone before objectively assessing the risks involved?	2	1	0
8. Do you lack close friends you can lean on if necessary?	2	1	0
9. Do you feel guilty about relaxing and enjoying life's pleasures (flower, poem, sky, etc.)?	2	1	0
10. Do you make your happiness conditional upon a person, event, or situation?	2	1	0
11. Do you want to be loved by everyone?	2	1	0
12. Are you afraid to start talking to a perfect stranger?	2	1	0
13. Do you find it hard to touch someone you love?	2	1	0
14. Do you engage in extramarital sex?	2	1	0
15. Is there an emotional barrier between you and your family?	2	1	0

SCORES   _____   _____   _____

TOTAL   _____

Personal Safety & Health Risks	Often	Sometimes	Rarely
1. Do you use habit forming drugs like heroin, cocaine, marijuana, or any hallucinogenic drugs?	5	3	0
2. Are you 20% over your ideal weight?	5	3	0
3. Do you have high cholesterol or triglycerides?	5	3	0
4. Do you smoke one pack per day or more of cigarettes?	5	3	0
5. Do you inhale or come into skin contact with dangerous chemicals in your job?	5	3	0
6. Would you jump right into some vigorous adventure sport without proper training and progression?	5	3	0

Personal Safety & Health Risks	Often	Sometimes	Rarely
7. Do you frequently handle or play with guns?	5	3	0
8. Do you participate in adventure sports like skydiving, hang-gliding, scuba diving, snowmobiling, mountain climbing, white water canoeing, auto racing, or similar sports?	5	3	0
9. Is your blood sugar markedly elevated (Diabetic) or markedly low (Hypoglycemic)?	5	3	0
10. Are you inactive, that is, sitting or standing at work and also at home?	5	3	0
11. Are you 10% over your ideal weight?	2	1	0
12. Do you use tranquilizers, pain relievers, antacid pills, or similar drugs?	2	1	0
13. Are you nervous, irritable, tense?	2	1	0
14. Do you experience insomnia and fatigue?	2	1	0
15. Do you spend your free time indoors?	2	1	0
16. Are you exposed to fluorescent lights?	2	1	0
17. Are you exposed to loud, irritating noises?	2	1	0
18. Do you live in an area of high air pollution?	2	1	0
19. Do you feel overcrowded?	2	1	0
20. Are you a weekend athlete (do nothing in between)?	2	1	0
21. Do you take the "pill"?			0
22. If you are in training for a specific event and you begin to experience frequent fatigue, insomnia, and lethargy, will you push yourself all the harder?	2	1	0
23. Females: I forget to examine my breasts for lumps at least once a month. Males: I forget to examine my testicles at least once a month.	2	1	0

SCORES _____ _____ _____

TOTAL _____

Self-Responsibility Risks	*Often*	*Sometimes*	*Rarely*
1. If there is somthing you want very much are you willing to steal it rather than work for it?	5	3	0
2. Do you have the attitude that your health is completely in the hands of your doctor?	5	3	0
3. Are your goals poorly defined, very vague, and general?	2	1	0
4. Do you feel an education (college, etc.) is not worth the effort?	2	1	0
5. Do you invest in high risk financial ventures (oil, etc.)?	2	1	0
6. Do you gamble at horses, cards, with slot machines, etc.?	2	1	0
7. Do you get more satisfaction from having acquired money rather than knowledge?	2	1	0
8. Do you see yourself as an incompetent person?	2	1	0
9. Do you enjoy pornographic movies, literature, games, etc.?	2	1	0
10. Do you spend your leisure time watching TV?	2	1	0
11. Do you drive without adequate liability insurance?	2	1	0
12. Do you have inadequate or no health insurance?	2	1	0
13. Do you buy things you can't really afford because you want to maintain a certain image?	2	1	0
14. As an investor do you put all your eggs in one basket rather than diversify (mutual funds, etc.)?	2	1	0
15. Do you invest time and money playing video computer games?	2	1	0

SCORES   _____   _____   _____

TOTAL   _____

Travel & Personal Safety Risks	Often	Sometimes	Never
1. Do you drink while driving?	5	3	0
2. Do you exceed the speed limits?	5	3	0
3. Do you fail to wear your seat belt and shoulder harness?	5	3	0
4. When you are mad or angry, do you take out your frustration behind the wheel?	5	3	0
5. Do you drive a motorcycle (weather permitting)?	5	3	0
6. Do you fail to wear a helmet when motorcycling or bicycling?	2	1	0
7. Do you have about one moving violation per year?	2	1	0
8. Is most of your driving in heavy traffic (urban vs. rural)?	2	1	0
9. Do you drive closely behind the driver in front of you (tailgating or trying to hurry him up)?	2	1	0
10. Do you drive more than 20 miles round trip to work?	2	1	0

SCORES _____ _____ _____

TOTAL _____

Nutritional Risks	Often	Sometimes	Rarely
1. Do you drink 4 or more cups of coffee per day (caffeinated or decaffeinated)?	5	3	0
2. Do you consume a high fat diet (foods like red meats, sausage, french fries, bacon, hot dogs, fried foods)?	5	3	0
3. Do you consume a high sugar diet (Foods like candy, pop, donuts, ice cream, pre-sweetened cereals, cookies, pies, cakes)?	5	3	0
4. Do you experiment with diet foods to lose weight (Atkin's Diet, Liquid Protein Diet, etc.)?	5	3	0

Nutritional Risks	Often	Sometimes	Rarely
5. Do you drink tap water?	2	1	0
6. Do you consume a high salt diet (canned vegetables, french fries, fast food meals, etc.)?	2	1	0
7. Do you eat highly processed foods instead of whole grain products (white bread, rolls, instant cereals, white rice, etc.)?	2	1	0
8. Do you omit fresh fruit and vegetables from your diet?	2	1	0
9. Do you use diet pills to curb your appetite?	2	1	0
10. Do you consume food containing nitrites and nitrates (used as a preventitive in hot dogs, beef jerky, bacon, some polish sausage, etc.)?	2	1	0
11. Do you drink more than one drink of hard liquor or 2 drinks of beer or wine daily?	2	1	0
12. Do you fail to take a high potency multiple vitamin mineral supplement on a daily basis?	2	1	0
SCORE	_____	_____	_____
TOTAL		_____	

Now add up each section to get your GRAND TOTAL. Compare it with the rating chart below to see how good a risk taker you are.

Grand Score	Rating	Comments
0–10	Superb	A rare person-return book and get your money back. Spread the wellness gospel.
11–25	Excellent	You should live long AND well with your risk-taking skills.
26–45	Good	Keep going-read the book to sharpen your skills.
46–70	Fair	You need to increase your awareness and wellness.
71–94	Poor	You are a daredevil-by all means read this book and, in the meantime, be sure the life insurance is paid.

Grand Score	Rating	Comments
95 +	Very Poor	You are also a daredevil-pray and prepare to meet your maker soon.

My current score on this questionnaire is 17 points, five of those because I take part in adventure sports, some of which I describe later in this section. Many of the risks you were asked about can kill you, either because you are accident prone or you are doing things that predispose you to cancer, heart disease, diabetes, stroke, or some other preventable disease. The boredom syndrome may be predisposing you to such diseases or accidents, and thus keeping you from reaching peak performance and enjoying life to the fullest.

Diagnosing Chronic Boredom

Clinicians or others who wish to utilize a scientifically validated instrument in diagnosing boredom should refer to an article by Jennifer Savitz, Ph.D, and Myles Friedman, Ph.D, "Diagnosing Boredom and Confusion," published in *Nursing Research* (Vol. 30 No. 1, Jan.-Feb. 1981).

How do *you* know if you're suffering from chronic boredom? Simple. Take this short test and find out.

1. Do you find yourself taking larger and larger quantities of stimulants (nicotine, caffeine, alcohol, marijuana, cocaine, tranquilizers, as well as food)?
2. Are you rarely excited and enthusiastic about life?
3. Do you frequently have problems finding things to keep you busy and interested?
4. Do you have very little control over how you spend your time each day?
5. Do you frequently spend more than three hours per day watching television?
6. Do you frequently feel tired and exhausted?

If you answered *yes* to more than two of these questions, chances are you're suffering from a sense of boredom, among other things. Perhaps the last question is the most telling. Adequate stimulation combats fatigue in a most interesting way. Through a phenomenon called *psycho-sensory restitution,* appropriate forms of stimulation can restore the nervous system's level of functioning to one of higher alertness, leaving a pleasant sensation of experiencing more of the world around us.

Too many of the same stimulus patterns (whether people, places, foods, or behaviors) create a feeling of fatigue and lethargy. This principle of psycho-sensory restitution was first demonstrated by Dr. Marta Grunewold, a music physiologist, using the pupillary reflex of the eye. With sophisticated recording equipment she found that the eye muscle would, with repetition of the same light stimulus, completely fail to respond after a relatively short time. Exhaustion had occurred. But, by simply interposing a new stimulus (sound), the experimenter could restore completely the eye muscle's response to the same light stimulus. As she stated:

> The individual, while awake, is constantly exposed to sensory and psychological stimuli. . . . Each of these stimuli, according to the principle of psycho-sensory restitution, can be expected to be constantly active in this sense of the principle, i.e., counteracting fatigue and exhaustion in all vegetative functions—a process which maintains the overall functioning capacity of the awake body.

Yes, variety of stimulation can prevent fatigue and too much monotony can cause it. The challenge is to find ways to create proper stimulation that is not detrimental to health and wellness. That is the aim of this book.

CHAPTER 1
Selected References

Alfredsson, Lars, and Tores Theorell. "Job Characteristics of Occupations and Myocardial Infarction Risk: Effect of Possible Confounding Factors." *Soc. Sci. & Medicine,* Vol. 17, No. 20, 1983.

Carney, Richard F. (ed.). *Risk Taking Behavior.* Charles C. Thomas, 1972.

Jougla, E., and others. "Health and Employment of a Female Population in an Urban Area." *Inter. Jour. of Epidemiology,* Vol. 12, No. 1, 1983.

Zuckerman, Marvin. *Sensation Seeking—Beyond the Optimal Level of Arousal.* Lea Publishing, 1979.

CHAPTER 2
The Doctor Is the Guinea Pig

How to deal with boredom seems to be the main issue in contemporary society, though few sociologists and even fewer psychologists readily admit it.

Some years ago I found my life had become too predictable. A pattern had begun to emerge, one which usually brought me full circle to my starting point. It went this way: Full of energy and enthusiasm, I'd launch myself into some new professional challenge—starting a rehabilitation center for heart patients in a city where none existed, starting a department of Wellness and Health Promotion in a hospital where none existed, or some similar project. Within six months the gears would be running smoothly. By the end of a year, progress always seemed to bring with it the full sprouting of a bureaucracy: more personnel, more compartmentalization of services, more uniformity, more rules, more committee meetings, and conferences on whether the bathroom door should read "Gentlemen" or just "Men." Individual initiative and new ideas soon became buried in paperwork or tossed about between menu selections (for tax writeoffs) during the more and more frequent "business lunches."

As conservatism and regimentation seem to be valued by many administrators, my enthusiasm would wane. The machines I helped build, though well oiled and showy, became cumbersome and slow, and walking with ankle weights is not my style. Boredom would soon set in. Soft chairs and walnut desks had lost their appeal as symbols of achievement.

So what does one do? There is, of course, a wide assortment of options; alcohol or marijuana to "mellow you out," cigarettes and caffeine to speed you up; sex and super-sex; food or other methods of compensation.

What I chose was none of those, but rather a three-year lifestyle that ranged from stuntman, to "mad scientist," to ultra-endurance athlete—in other words, exploring danger, researching risks, and dabbling in the psychology of extreme sports. During that three-year period, I participated in stunt-car driving, scuba diving, skydiving, downhill skiing, mountain motocross, white-water canoeing, swimming down dangerous rivers, flying an ultra-light (a motorized hang glider), cliff diving, bridge jumping,

15

rock climbing, and building climbing (the sport known officially as "buildering"). Some of these I will describe shortly.

If a poor man engages in bizarre forms of behavior, we label him "crazy," if a rich man does so we label him "eccentric"; those in between are often just called "deviates." I became a deviate. (More than likely I always was one.) Oh well, at least I had had respectability for a while, but now I'd come out of the closet. It happened innocently enough. There I was one evening watching television and drinking a beer, and there went a car flying off an embankment into a lake. *That would be fun,* I thought— to perform that stunt, to experience the sensation of flying through the air in an automobile knowing that the heavy shell would take the impact and protect you from harm. I only toyed with the idea, not really intending to do the thing. But, curiosity has a funny way of teasing one's arousal level. The married person who suspects an attractive member of the opposite sex desires him or her creates situations to test those beliefs, and heightens the arousal level in the process.

As I gained more information, did more research, and talked to race car drivers and Hollywood stuntmen (who initially tried to dissuade me), I began to believe it could be done safely, that it could be, like the roller coaster, a controlled risk. I also found that it was an excellent antidote for the boredom and frustrations I was experiencing from nine to five. It was, after all, something I had complete control of, an event which, assuming I took every possible precaution, could be a lot of fun. "The prospect of the gallows," as one writer said, "does much to sharpen the senses."

After some six months of planning and meticulous preparation, I made the jump, rode a car I'd purchased for a hundred dollars out over a six-foot embankment at thirty- five miles per hour into a lake. I remained in the car until it sank eighteen feet to the lake floor before I escaped.

There was no fanfare, no audience—just a well-selected crew of professional divers and equipment on hand to handle all the contingencies of the situation. All went smoothly; all exactly as planned.

Actually to have done this thing—to have plummeted through the air, nosedived into deep water and popped back up like a cork, survived the rapid descent to the silt bottom to be gently bounced along in slow motion—remains impregnated upon my senses to this day. Merely by closing my eyes and willing the experience back to mind, I recall that experience in every vivid detail as you will forever remember in detail the euphoric feelings on the day you rode your bicycle unassisted.

Initially it was to be an isolated event, certainly not one of a series, certainly not the subject matter of a book on risk taking. But as I reflected upon the stunt in its entirety, upon my preparation both mentally and physically, upon my motives for performing the stunt, many insights and ideas that presented themselves had relevance for wellness, safety, and success.

First and foremost was the notion of *self-responsibility,* that human beings are *not* merely straws carried by whatever wind currents find them and deposit them at random upon a thousand different surfaces. No, I was alive because I had used my mind to its fullest, had researched the risks and anticipated the possible outcomes. I had asked the experts what to expect, how to prepare myself. For example, the stuntmen I talked to were adamant in insisting I become a certified scuba diver in order to learn how to prevent my eardrums from breaking during my descent. Many other suggestions and advice were carefully followed. Yes, I had to assume self-responsibility for my own survival, learn wherein the risks lay and systematically go about eliminating them one by one until it was a safe adventure.

Closely tied to self-responsibility is the notion of "back-up systems," or secondary plans, just in case something goes wrong with your primary plan. For example, although I had practiced breath-holding exercises until I could hold my breath four and one half minutes, nevertheless I took *two* scuba tanks with me to the bottom. One was fastened just to my right on the passenger's seat and one was securely fastened behind my own seat with a breathing regulator coming directly over my shoulder. Once in the water I inserted it in my mouth so I had an ample supply of air at all times. This procedure was recommended by the stuntmen I talked to.

In addition to the primary back-up system, the professional divers (with their tanks) would be nearby within seconds after my submersion just in case, even prepared to cut me out of the car if necessary. (Many cars turn upside down during submersion because of the air in the tires.)

In short, I was prepared for any unforeseen mishap using such back-up systems, a concept of great relevance, which will be discussed again later.

Second, the notion of *safety,* one essential component of wellness, maximizing personal safety through good control of the environment, the equipment, and the quality of experience. All accidents and mishaps can be traced to a filure to anticipate problems in one of those three areas.

In the car stunt, I wore the five-point safety harness used in race cars. It held me securely and prevented my body from being thrown about in any direction. Also, every possible modification to the car was made consistent with safety (bolting the hood down, welding the door shut, etc.) Even the gas tank was removed from the car to prevent a possible explosion. To provide a fuel source, a one-gallon gas container was fastened to the firewall with a line running to the fuel pump.

The third implication for wellness was *stress management:* how to relax and achieve my goal, namely survival. Physical fitness, nutrition, visualization, learning to think creatively, and proper mental attitude all played a valuable role in this regard. But the technique that worked best was a combination of running for relaxation, combined with the use of visualization. To use the visualization technique effectively, however, one must actually become one with the event and the environment in which the event unfolds. To do so requires a somewhat metaphysical way of looking at life because it means attributing characteristics of living beings to inanimate objects or nonliving substance and materials.

For example, in the stunt described, water was not just water, with a certain temperature, specific gravity (density), and color. No, it became much more. It became a substance that softened the impact by cradling me in its arms and rocking me gently back and forth until the forces had dissipated. "Personification", the association with positive emotions of caring, loving, and trust were of immense help in remaining relaxed and at peace while performing a stunt of such potential danger. More on this technique later.

Finally, I was discovering my *uniqueness*. Insofar as these extreme sports and stunts seemed to fulfill a deep need in me, my research into risk taking (as well as the human risk-taking drive) also helped me understand this need. As I found, the human need for stimulation is strongly determined by our genetic makeup. Scientific studies have found that such needs vary widely among people. While some individuals can easily tolerate a mundane lifestyle, others go quietly insane, or drink or smoke themselves into oblivion in order to cope.

In order to learn more about my own need system as well as to document any personality changes that might occur as the result of such continued activities, I requested extensive testing by Dr. Don Vest, a psychologist at Washburn University. In order to shed light on the direction my lifestyle had suddenly taken, I took a battery of six different tests, including Dr. Marvin Zuckerman's Sensation Seeking Scale. The result?

> Dr. Crookse scores extremely high on needs for aggression, autonomy, and achievement. Test scores as well as interviews show him not to be foolish or foolhardy but rather to demonstrate very high needs for thrill and adventure seeking, and markedly high scores on boredom susceptibility. . . . These needs are somewhat actualized in hs desire for high risk activities.

The greatest discovery is oneself. Recall that uniqueness is a vital component of high-level wellness. This is perhaps the greatest risk of all, deviating from the norm, leaving your comfort zone, to develop the characteristics or talents that differentiate you from others. The tests had merely confirmed what I had come to recognize instinctively while pursuing that car stunt: that I had a profound need to be testing myself in some manner or fashion involving extreme sports and stunts. I'd experienced a great deal of personal learning about concepts I'd only read about in sports psychology books. And where there is lots of growth and self-discovery, there can be no boredom.

I decided to continue my "wellness experiments" to further test my theories first hand. In the chapter that follows, I will briefly describe five more such endeavors.

CHAPTER 3

Stunts and Extreme Sports as Wellness Experiments

The Odyssey was Homer's epic poem describing Ulysses' ten-year wanderings while returning home to Ithaca after the Trojan War. Ulysses wanted to test himself, to gain great wisdom by overcoming obstacles and severe challenges. His colorful adventures provided the all-important stimulation so necessary to feeling fully alive. He invoked his fellow mariners:

> How dull it is to pause, to make an end, to rest unburnished, not to shine in use . . . you were not formed to live like brutes but to follow virtue and knowledge.

As a graduate student I'd taken many courses in the psychology of sport and physical activity. But books without personal experience are like cars without wheels. The real test of one's theories is not within the sterile confines of a laboratory but in the daily flow of life. We call this concept experiential learning. It was time for some experiential learning; it was time to have some fun.

Jumping to Conclusions from a 90-foot Bridge

Analysis of Risk Factors   In all my experiments following the car stunt I would first examine the stunt in detail; that is, break it down into its component parts in order to better understand the risk factors or variables that could kill me. In most cases I contacted Harvey Parry, a Hollywood stuntman of some fifty years experience. Harvey and I have had many conversations since our initial visit and it was during such conversations that I came to understand how these risk-factors for a stunt are quite identical to risk factors for a disease or illness. In both cases, one becomes aware of the variables, the behaviors or objects, that can escalate the likelihood of personal harm and injury.

Each risk factor for this 90-foot-bridge jump into the Missouri River was carefully analyzed: the height, the entry speed (63 mph), the poor visibility of the water and possibility of objects below the surface, and the fear of the water itself.

In each case, safety precautions were taken. I made hundreds of practice jumps beginning at 20 feet to perfect the correct technique, wearing a wetsuit to provide one-quarter-inch neoprene cushion around my body. I consulted with the Army Corps of Engineers on speed of the water and various depths under the bridge. Finally, I spent hours and hours swimming across and down the river. During my initial few swims I was tethered by a safety line to a boat to ensure I wouldn't be sucked under by some of the whirlpools and tricky currents that characterize the Missouri River.

Although local authorities weren't wild about my request to perform this stunt, as it turned out they had no choice, as the following letter from the city attorney stated:

> Dear Dr. Crookse:
>
> I have thoroughly reviewed our ordinances and found none that forbid jumping off a bridge. I talked to the police attorney and he indicated that the police wouldn't take you to The Psychiatric Receiving Center for an examination if it was clear that this wasn't necessary. In that connection, he indicated that if you wished to meet with him after your plans are firm, he'd make arrangements to have the officers patroling the area of the bridge informed of the circumstances of the jump.

Use of Visualization   To succeed in any major enterprise, you must believe in your goal so powerfully that you see it happening in your mind's eye. The following excerpt from my preparatory notes will give you an idea how I used this technique to survive my jump, how I tried to personify the bridge to give it its own sense of being and aliveness, and how I tried to associate pleasant happy thoughts with the bridge much as you would someone you loved and cared about.

> Coming back home from the KCI Airport, I had to pass over the bridge again. As I approached it heading south toward downtown Kansas City late in the evening, I realized for the first time what a beautiful bridge it really was, not just a long flat concrete slab like many of the modern bridges. No, it was cable supported, like the larger Golden Gate Bridge in San Francisco, with swaying cables draped from one support to the other. This gentle curvature created the effect of cathedral spires laced together like Gothic architecture. I pulled over to the shoulder of the Interstate to admire this wondrous looking structure. It was that time of evening when, like a Christmas tree coming to life, the lights of the city suddenly turn on in full color and your mood heightens, buoyed up by the prospect of nightlife and romance. The red beacon lights atop the spires came on and I thought, "How could something so lovely provoke such fear?" But right here at this moment, there was no fear, for the bridge became as a beautiful woman, opening her arms toward me and beckoning me forward. From that time on, I never called it a bridge

again. I thought of her as a woman, she was feminine, she was life, she was love and she could never hurt me once I understood her mysteries. This kind of association emotionally relaxed me, I became one with something which normally exists only in the physical plane. "Isn't she beautiful?" I always thought whenever I approached her. "She's beautiful, she's magnificent. She's nothing to fear. She is only to be understood."

Another bit of information taken from my journal describes how visualization contributed to my success in this dangerous stunt:

> Later in the week I located my jump spot, just about ten feet south of one of the bridge supports, since that's where the water was deepest. Now I could begin to visualize myself jumping from the bridge. I took the bridge photos and had them enlarged. Then, I cut out photos taken while jumping at lower heights and overlaid them onto the bridge photos in such a way that it looked as though I was jumping from the bridge. I integrated this picture into my mind until it became an entire motion picture sequence. You should see the images in vivid detail, using every one of your senses. I'd spend my lunch hour sitting below the bridge to get the "feel" of the whole environment, closing my eyes and listening to the cars overhead, the gurgle of water against the sharp rocks, the faucet like sound of water rushing on either side of the huge bridge supports, and the occasional whistle of a tugboat downstream. I had to become part of this environment and it had to become a part of me, even the poignant odor of the river, which smelled like a dead carcass. We'd become one till the challenge was met.
>
> The picture began to take form in my mind, and I began to imagine jumping from the bridge many times each day and run this thought projection through my mind in slow motion sometimes stopping at certain frames to make corrections in my form.

And the jump itself? That I had programmed my mind so well probably saved me from disaster, because that one-in-a-thousand freak occurrence happened. At precisely the moment I jumped, an eighteen-wheeler whizzed behind me on the bridge creating a wind blast; it propelled me forward with such momentum I was too far forward. But, my computer program locked in. I made the necessary adjustments in form and let the speed carry me to the water. I had landed well. I had managed the odds and survived my second rites of passage.

The Issue of Control I was alive thanks to God *and* Mark. I had managed the risks, used my mind and body to the fullest, ate well, and ran to resolve the tension. I even ran three miles just prior to the jump itself. So as I think about other peoples' lives, I think about the smaller, less intense though perhaps more lethal risks they take, and I wonder how prepared they are.

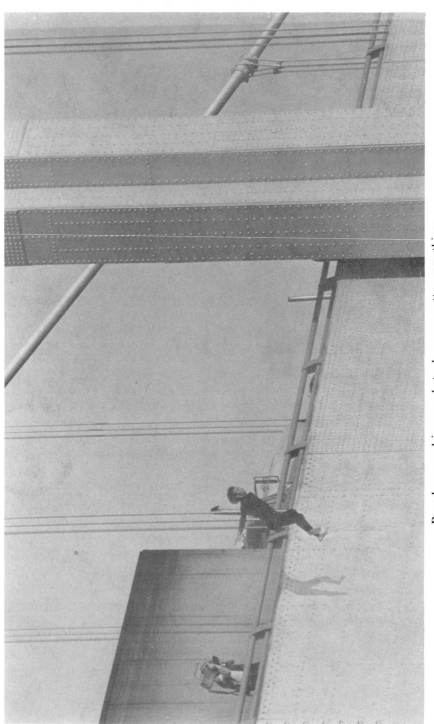

Boredom can drive people to do some pretty crazy things.

Swimming to St. Louis

Analysis of Risk Factors By now, I had become the center of much media attention. While this recognition can be a positive thing, it can also create its own hazards and risk factors because now you begin to realize others will sit in judgment of your performance. Such awareness can be distracting and create stresses beyond the demands of the feat itself. As is often seen in high level athletes however, you must learn to handle such stress to make it work for you, rather than against you. World records are not set during practice, but during the stress of competition, under the scrutiny of larger audiences who share vicariously in the performance. In sports psychology, we call this increased arousal and activation level created by an audience *social facilitation.*

Three front-page stories on the bridge jump and my attempt to swim and body float 375 miles down the Missouri River to St. Louis created a great deal of pressure. My best insurance for success was to be physically in superb condition.

Other risk factors included snakes, whirlpools, large fish (channelcat and sturgeon can weigh over 100 lbs.), and barges that were a definite safety hazard. But perhaps the risk factor of greatest concern was the water temperature. Delays had pushed me into October and water temperature of 60 degrees can quickly produce *hypothermia* (lowered body temperature). Hypothermia can cause sensory depression, abnormal heart rhythms, unconsciousness, and if exposure continues, even death.

Exercise and Nutrition Effective management of risk factors required the use of a wetsuit to help reduce heat loss, frequent coatings of a mixture composed of Vaseline and lanolin, and the gradual increase of my exposure time in cold water—this last to condition myself mentally and physically for the cold stress involved. Since lowered body temperature can create a tremendous drain on one's resources, I also trained by running and swimming until I felt in peak condition. After all, this could mean the difference between life and death.

My diet was simple yet effective: focus on high-energy foods and complex carbohydrates like brown rice, dried fruit such as raisins, dates, and figs, and whole-grain breads, avoid junk food, and try to avoid red meats and other high-fat foods. According to the best estimates I could calculate, I'd be burning about 8,000 calories per day, and frequent small feedings of fruits, fruit juices, and pasta helped me maintain a high, steady energy level. As we'll see later in the book, this pattern of frequent feedings of high fiber foods helps regulate insulin levels. (In many cases it can control diabetes more effectively than drugs.) In addition, once a day I received an intravenous infusion of vitamin C (25 grams) and minerals administered by a physician friend who had conducted much research on vitamin C and stress. This seemed to aid my adaptation to the severe cold.

Since I breaststroked most of the time while being carried in the currents of the main channel (to avoid whirlpools), I ate my meals on a styrofoam tray, which bounced about on the water's surface. Occasionally, waves created by passing barges would send me chasing after my meal as it headed toward shore.

Stress Management Most of us have no idea what we can accomplish until pushed to the limit. Were it not for the fact that I felt pressure from all the media coverage, I probably would have quit on the afternoon of the first day, the cold became so uncomfortable. Indeed, the highlight of my day was urinating in my wetsuit and luxuriating in the warm flow which traveled up and surrounded my midsection. It was a contentment the reader may not understand, may even find disgusting. But there simply comes a time, a suffering threshhold, when one sets aside the established rules of conduct in order to survive as easily as possible. Twenty hours a day I breast stroked and floated, for nearly seven consecutive days, enjoying the warmth of sunlight provided by an Indian Summer while at night receding into myself, to renew my psychic energies, meditate, and study the constellations that dotted my nighttime ceiling.

Most of the barges slowed when they saw the light of the pontoon boat that accompanied me. Several times we heard the river warnings over the marine radio:

> A swimmer will leave Kansas City from LaBenite Park on Sept. 27th and will be in the water at night. Please be on the watch. He will be heading for St. Louis, expecting to arrive on the fourth of October. He will be accompanied by a pontoon boat.

A passing tugboat sent us a message: "Hope your guy makes it. He must be awfully cold."

There was always a powerful mood change at sunset. The sun slipped below the horizon, producing a sense of awe at the mirror images of gold, orange, and purple upon the water. Then, as I began to meditate to dissociate myself from my cold surroundings, I discovered a most remarkable thing. Once I entered the "void," where all incoming thoughts and present reality are filtered out, my shivering would stop. If someone broke my trancelike state, the shivering would resume. Once I discovered such control over my situation, my outlook became very positive. I became more and more adept at meditating in this fashion during the cold quiet of nighttime.

Games and play can be effective means of reducing feelings of distress. Racing for beers that rode on styrofoam boats and throwing tennis balls at each other as we floated downriver served as diversions for the mind. (We'd taken 200 tennis balls to throw at various points in the river's width to find the fastest currents).

Taking time to appreciate the simple elegancies of life also helps one keep things in perspective. Environmental awareness helps one enjoy the trip as well as the arriving. As written in my journal:

> By now we began to see more and more bluffs extending high above the river. Caves, cut deep into limestone rocks, took us back to an earlier time. We imagined an indian emerging from a cave to watch his intruders pass by. The wildlife we saw consisted of an occasional beaver in the gray of early morning or late evening swimming for cover, or an egret, tip-toeing among the marshes on his stilt legs, and lots of geese landing on the sand beaches to feed enroute to their warm winter habitat. They moved busily back and forth, filling the air with their cackling sounds, and poking at the sand for edibles of some kind.
>
> Many of these beaches, or sandbars, isolated from people, stretched white and clean as new sandpaper along the shallow side of the river for almost a mile. I often tried to walk onto one, only to find myself standing on the edge of a sandbar, then pushed over a dropoff by the current. This uncertain footing made me fearful as I wasn't sure if river quicksand was myth or reality. I left this beauty to the geese.

Environmental awareness means being sensitive to changing times, and to people caught in the midst of such changes. The Gasconade River empties into the Missouri ninety miles upstream from St. Louis. Once emerald green and pure because of its underground springs, it now flowed brown with yet a tint of its former self. At a riverside park while getting supplies I found out why. Walter told me why. He was one of those sun parched, weathered relics every small rivertown has, a walking testimony of bygone days when life moved as lazily as the river did during that unseasonably dry summer. He said, "All started when they tore the God-damn outhouses down! No more damn fish, big'uns anyhow."

Walter, standing there in his fishline stitched coveralls, smelling of dried bait, and dribbling brown juice out the corner of his mouth from his chewin' tobacco had just given me his version of a complex social change, but it had a certain truth. For then came modern waste disposal, chemical water treatment, sewage systems dumping into rivers, rivers too dirty to swim.

Goals and Supergoals Setting your sights high and aiming for lofty pinnacles is fine, but climb in increments. Be philosophical about life, be patient, and (though not forgetting the larger goal) take one day at a time. Time is not your adversary in wellness medicine, it is your ally; it sprouts thoughts and waters the tree of wisdom. Otherwise the magnitude of mountain tops can overwhelm you. This was the philosophy I adopted, setting smaller objectives, focusing on getting around the next bend, or reaching the next town.

The days melted together with but a few respites in between, but at 5:00 P.M. on the seventh day I finally spotted the Gateway Arch towering majestically above the St. Louis skyline, itself a symbol of risk takers, pioneers who pursued their dreams.

I felt euphoric, even heroic. I'd accomplished something I once considered nearly impossible. I'd found a system for success; You set high goals (relative to *your* present ability in some area), you identify and manage the risks enroute to that goal, you apply wellness principles of peak performance, and you'll finish a winner.

Epilogue   It is a year later to the day now, as I sit here ever so solemnly on the river bank and watch the brown sudsy water flow by. Some day I'll bring my son or daughter down here. We'll sit on this same river bank and discuss the river, and talk about risking. They'll experience a deeper life. They too will try.

Two-Day Submersion

The idea of remaining underwater for one day, maybe even longer, always fascinated me, I mean wondering what it would be like psychologically without the normal diversions of telephones, television, automobiles, and all the other toys we use to occupy ourselves. What would happen under those circumstances, cut off from sensory stimulation, what kind of psychological tunnel does one go through and where are the exits, the passageways of the mind that keep one sane under such states of isolation and confinement?

Maximizing Safety   Of course, there were the risk factors to consider; prolonged exposure to chlorine, the fatigue associated with loss of sleep, holding a mouthpiece in place, and the possibility of balance problems and ear infections. But these could be easily resolved. The psychological risks? That was another story.

As I researched and gathered material on sensory deprivation, I found that this kind of submersion could produce about every psychological disorder listed in the *Manual of Psychological Disorders*. For example, subjects in one study became paranoid, or disoriented; many began to hallucinate in uncontrollable ways. Other findings indicated that many people would report out-of-body experiences or extreme irritability and restlessness. Lethargy, depression, and eventually anxiety could become so severe that the most "macho" of men were often transformed into trembling, feeble-looking creatures. Also, because a time distortion often occurred, people would lose touch with reality, for time structures our life; it provides the framework for our activities; it is the pendulum and chime that signals a change in behavior.

To survive prolonged submersion requires a strong, stable personality, someone who likes himself or herself and is happy with life, because the stress of prolonged submersion quickly peels away the superficial layers of one's personality and exposes the underlying self. People with an immature ego, or weak personality, who are ego-defensive, don't last long under such conditions, as my research suggested.

Stress Management　How would I deal with all of this? The first law of survival is fitness, being in the best possible condition, having high energy levels that translate to high frustration tolerance. Diet and fitness were maximized. But there were other ploys, other wellness tools to draw upon. One of these was *subliminal communication*. That strange word simply means communicating with someone *below* the level of conscious detection; in other words, at the level of the subconscious. Subliminal communication first gained notoriety when used in a New Jersey motion picture theatre to promote sales of popcorn and Coca-Cola. Here's how it worked. Periodically during the movie, a frame with a picture of popcorn or Coca-Cola would be interjected in such a way that, although the conscious mind did not detect the single frame, the subconscious "saw" the isolated frame. Then, the person would think, *I'm hungry for some popcorn*, or *I'm thirsty for some Coke*. Sales went up considerably. Once the media got wind of such mind-control techniques, there was a large-scale reaction and these techniques were quickly halted. But subliminal communication is being used by some researchers to enhance wellness; that is, for weight control, enhancing motivation, improving sports performance, smoking cessation, and reducing shoplifting.

Dr. Hal Becker of the Behavioral Engineering Institute in Metairie, Louisiana, is one of the leading authorities in this area. Hal agreed to help program my subconscious mind with such affirmative statements as, "I am healthy, my ears are healthy, nothing can harm them, my immune system protects me from anything, my ears are bacteria free, my balance is perfect, I am in control, I am strong." These messages, embedded in music and played on underwater speakers, would help me manage the stresses of isolation and confinement.

Other stress-management techniques I planned to use included meditation, proper use of lighting, touching (if necessary), and the use of a habitat to create a feeling of safety (shelter). Most of these ideas were developed following a trial submersion of nearly twenty hours. As it turned out, I remained underwater for two entire days. The following observations were taken from my journal and should give you some idea of how and why the techniques described were used.

> The pool was 25' by 40' and I discovered "the fish bowl effect," meaning that everything within those confines is soon viewed, touched, or otherwise explored and there remains nothing to do but swim periodic circles around the pool walls. By the sixth hour, I had memorized every miniature crater formed by the excessive hydrochloric acid in the pool water. So what do you do, perform somersaults, and other forms of play? Still, eventually boredom catches you.
>
> I learned to have sympathy for the obese person who eats his way through

life, living from meal to meal with fantasies of food. I was drinking liquid meals provided through plastic containers, an idea obtained from the Space Craft Center in Houston, and used to prevent bowel movements while astronauts were in space. I soon tired of this liquid meal and began to dwell more and more on chocolate pudding, strawberry shortcake, ice cream, and apple strudel. See, when boredom becomes severe enough, even junk food sounds great.

You must be as the philosopher, as the deep thinker, to remain submerged this long because this becomes your only escape, to the inner recesses of your mind, to search the memory for pieces of information lost amid the maelstrom of daily life.

But you soon discover the infinite magnitude of the human memory, all the creative thoughts, and unresolved conclusions. I'd relive an entire segment of my life and find that time flew by. Sometimes I'd meditate for hours on end, going back into the forgotten files and video tapes of my memory and gathering additional insights into events, situations, and people and see my life not as the participant but as the spectator. This provided the stimulation I needed. Sometimes I'd just find the void, completely let go become nonexistent, suspended somewhere between life and death, falling indefinitely without speed or fear of impact.

As I achieved such states, my metabolic rate would drop enormously and air tanks which once lasted two hours now lasted five or six, and divers observing me would occasionally come down and rouse me to awareness to assure themselves of my safety. I had become an underwater yogi.

One observation from my trial submersion had been how quickly I became depressed when denied light of the proper intensity in my underwater home. As research at the National Institutes of Health and elsewhere has shown, light strongly affects our emotions. Some patients have had their depressed moods altered simply by regulating the type, duration, and intensity of light. Light is even being used to enhance the immune system and treat a wide variety of disorders from jet lag to insomnia. Again, from my journal:

My most enjoyable experience with lights occurred between 1:00 and 4:00 p.m. when lots of natural daylight would come pouring through the motel's skylights located above the pool and light up two large cubes below the water's surface. I was attracted to these light sources and spent most of the time between those hours basking in this natural light. I couldn't help but reflect upon the fact, in our hurried and confined lifestyles we've cut ourselves off from the natural light we need. Scientists are just now beginning to realize the side effects of artificial light, especially low-spectrum fluorescent lighting. These include hyperactivity, decreased calcium absorption, and loss of hair.

Shelter   This has a strong psychological impact upon our lives though we often take it for granted. During the trial submersion I'd experienced a profound sense of vulnerability, of being "watched" by unknown eyes. But a habitat constructed of fiberglass panels resolved some of that previous distress. It provided a feeling of safety, of security. In researching this matter, I found that fear of wide-open, exposed spaces is inborn in Homo Sapiens. Most inborn fears had strong evolutionary value. When primitive man found himself fully exposed and remote from any place to hide, he was more vulnerable to his enemies, wild animals, or the elements. Perhaps, during the previous submersion, this instinctive fear was uncovered. At any rate, I felt this drive to return to the habitat periodically grow more potent as the time passed by.

Touching, Loving, Hugging The most profound observation associated with this experiment occurred about 1:00 A.M. of the first night. The feeling of isolation just overwhelmed me. I informed the attending psychologist that I was ready to end the experiment. But Dr. Becker quickly perceived the problem and instructed Vickie, my fiancée, to jump into the water and begin rubbing my neck. What a miracle drug, this human touch. Within thirty seconds the sense of fear was completely gone. As my research later uncovered, touch therapy is used in holistic medicine to enhance our immune system, increase energy levels in sick people, and make us more resistant to numerous diseases. I never experienced anxiety or fear again from then on.

Issue of Control Boredom is a very powerful force which molds much of our behaviours. Stimulation is absolutely necessary but we can maintain control by selecting those behaviors and thoughts which promote self-reliance.

Ironically, it is possible to be stimulation-hungry in the midst of crowds and rush-hour traffic. For what is a highly regimented, unchallenging job but another version of a sensory deprivation chamber? Yet, under the most sensory deprived of situations we still have at our disposal a powerful wellness tool, meditation, and the nearly infinite maze of psychic corridors that remain unexplored. We should periodically retreat to those corridors, to get alone for awhile, and perhaps even experience a sense of loneliness. Then, touch, light, colors, and the sounds of nature will become magnified in their effects, rather than forgotten in our search for superstimuli.

Epilogue Some years back, I'd hidden a twenty-dollar bill for a special purpose and had long forgotten where I put it. While underwater I remembered where it was. Upon returning home, sure enough, I found it in Max Maultz's book, *Psycho-Cybernetics,* Chapter 13, "How to Turn A Crisis Into A Creative Opportunity."

The First-Time Skydive—a 9000-foot Freefall

Jumping out of an airplane—opening the door of a flying projectile 12,000 feet high and throwing your body into midair—defies survival instincts innate to man over thousands of evolutionary years. Man hunted and was hunted for eons; he came to understand the fear of attack from enemies and wild beasts as part of the life scheme. He understood the darkness as a time to rest and as a hiding place for those who wished him harm. He understood the fear of moving water but also learned to harness it. He learned early in life, by ever-so-delicate lessons, that falling is painful. Even the young baby who develops upright locomotion won't venture forth from a shallow ledge.

Considering these natural fears, it is not surprising that only eighty years ago, a tiny fraction of man's natural history, has man had the advantage of human flight. And consider further the totally unnatural act of falling through space with no reference point beyond the sounds of air screaming by your ears, like the Sirens of Circe's drawing you toward self-destruction.

Is it any wonder then that so many people cannot learn to override this fear, to suppress all the rational thoughts which suggest certain suicide? But then, this is all the more reason to do it, to gain the greater perspective upon yourself, to grow beyond the limits to which fear restricts you.

Analysis of Risk Factors   As in all aspects of wellness medicine, the hazards to health and safety must be assessed. In this experiment, the most obvious was the experience factor—learning the correct technique for leaving the plane, falling correctly, deploying the parachute, and landing (broken ankles are common). Weather variables are of prime consideration since novice jumpers increase their risk of mishaps if conditions aren't optimal. Strong winds have killed or injured many skydivers. State-of-the-art equipment also maximizes safety, since in the newer parachutes, less time and effort is required to deploy a reserve chute should a malfunction occur. High-quality training, using audiovisual devices and cockpit mockups, can also contribute measurably to the safety margin.

But, as in all of my experiments, extreme as they were, psychological preparation was my greatest concern, especially since this was not to be a typical first-time jump.

I'd already received special permission from the U.S. Parachute Association to freefall for one mile on my first attempt. The usual procedure is to use a "static line," which opens the chute automatically ten feet out of the plane. For one full minute I'd freefall earthward, to experience my body in flight and collect some medical data as well. I planned to take blood chemistries and EKGs during the actual freefall, using a special twenty-four-hour monitoring package attached to my waist. I was required to undergo a rigorous training program (Accelerated Freefall School), and submit any findings to the U.S.P.A.

Back-Up Systems   Remember once more, managing risks effectively requires back-up systems. In this case, not only did I wear a reserve chute (an absolute must!) but I wore an automatic opener, a pressure/speed-sensitive device that, activated by a 22 rifle shell, fires the reserve chute if someone is so paralyzed by fear they "freeze." In addition, two representatives from the U.S.P.A. would train and jump with me, to be ready to offer assistance if safety required it.

Visualization The following passages from my journal will give you an idea how I used this wellness technique to overcome the fears;

> I cut out pictures of skydivers from skydiving magazines, many with aerial photos depicting the earth below them or the blue sky in the background. I mounted a great many of these on large poster boards so I could spend many hours viewing them while listening to relaxing music. I wanted to think like the skydiver, fill my mind with perceptual information as he experiences it, to become one with the sport as much as was possible. We, in our earthbound existence, always perceive the world from the horizontal, but rarely straight down. But, I quickly recognized the importance of feeding into my visual field the earth from upside down if I was to relax while falling at speeds of 120 mph toward earth.
>
> Another visualization technique involved the use of video tapes taken from a helmet mounted camera during actual skydives. I viewed this footage many times and began to memorize these images and replay them mentally during times of quiet relaxation.

The more I began to analyze the fear, as I certainly did many times, the more I began to understand it. It was *not* a fear of heights, it was *not* the fear of flying, it was *not* the fear of falling. It was a fear of the *unknown,* of entering a foreign world for one whole minute where there is nothing solid to hold onto, where the only reality which exists is the parachute on your back and the altimeter on your chest counting down the feet between you and the ground.

To supplement the visualization techniques, I took a series of five observation flights to watch the skydivers actually leave the plane. The last one of these was a 4th-of-July special, a nude skydive. I'd heard some wild stories about couples who engaged in petting and kissing while falling at 120 mph, but the nude skydive will never be forgotten. As written in my journal:

> By the time we reached 7,000 feet my ribs were sore from laughter. I watched their tanned bodies and sheet-white buttocks move onto the wing and sail away. Joining hands, they formed a star and as their bodies grew tiny, began to resemble three tiny babies frolicking and kicking, excited by the feel of grass on their tummies and the heat of the sun on their shiny white bottoms. In the midst of such laughter, my fears dissolved.

Fitness and Stress Management Running was the tranquilizer that always dispelled any anxiety. Often I'd run down the unused runways at the airport, out into pastures and farmlands that made up the drop zone. Running in the location of my fears while imagining myself falling through the sky in the jumper's arch always brought the blood pressure down to normal and left me in a positive mood. I cannot emphasize this enough.

The Malfunction   After four months of careful preparation, including intensive classroom instruction and practical training I made the jump. The following account of this jump taken from my journal describes what happened;

Around we go, banking steadily in circles, gaining altitude each time as I watch telephone poles become smeared dots, trees shrink into bushes and the earth become a giant checkerboard of brown and green squares. An occasional car, looking more like a tiny bug, runs along the perimeter of several squares. 6,000 feet. It's cold because the temperature drops 3.5° each thousand feet higher we go and as I look down again I notice an intriguing phenomenon produced by a thin haze of clouds, that all the browns and greens are fading into cold gray color. Every now and then, the Cessna 150 banks at a sharp angle and the sun's reflection off the larger ponds bounces back at me.

12,000 feet. The door was thrown open, I shifted my body out into the windblast and clasped the wingstrut. My jumpsuit snapped and popped as it whipped about in the 80 mph windblast. Out I plummeted, tumbling as in a dryer, flared my arms and legs and found the arched position, facing earth with the Missouri River snaking below me. A thousand air pressure fingers poked at me, jostled me about my center point (center of gravity) as I felt the airstream rush between my fingerspread. Shrill wind-sounds whistled through my helmet, magnifying the perception of speed. I was the willing participant in a magnificent display of body/brain feedback loops, each slight imbalance triggering a reflex corrective movement in the opposite arm or leg.

A mile zoomed by as though in seconds and it was time to pull the ripcord. . . . Nothing . . . another 2000 feet passed by and yet, there was not the least anxiety, just the rapture of the ride, the hypnotic free suspension on an airpressure column. 'Look up!', one of my companions motioned several times. As I later learned an air pressure vacuum, created by my wide shoulders, had trapped the pilot chute, dragging it uninflated next to my back until, looking behind me, the vacuum was spoiled by the airstream. This happens one in 2000 times but it has happened to me . . . Suddenly, total silence, and a slow motion sequence as I found myself sailing over the lush farmlands below. I'd been hurled through a screaming time tunnel machine and thrown into the quiet tranquility of the present on a warm July day. I had jumped beyond the door which held me prisoner, I felt more in control of life.

Epilogue   The stress of a first-time skydive caused no abnormal changes on my EKG, however a disagreement with my fiancée the same evening caused skips to appear in my heart rhythm when the EKG tapes were later scanned. A novice skydiving friend jumped a few months later in subzero temperatures. She was not wearing an automatic opener. She chose to ignore the rules of safety. She risked poorly, she died.

Climbing for Wellness—Up a Life Insurance Building

Life insurance companies gamble on your life. They gamble you'll survive long enough to pay the premiums. They consider themselves experts in risk management because they easily win at this game. In truth, they know very little about risk management. Financially, they succeed though. What's their secret?

Their secret is numbers, large numbers. They insure enough people so they can distribute their losses evenly among policyholders since they know how many people of any age, race, and sex will die each year. Thus, we all pay high premiums, and the well people reimburse the insurance companies for losses incurred on the sick people. This isn't risk management, this is death management. Many life insurance companies give lip service to health promotion, but few do anything to reward it. (A few do give reductions for those who stay fit.)

Uniqueness Factor   Climbing buildings seemed to be in vogue and it would be another good test of my risk taking theories. Sure, I could have gone off and climbed a mountain somewhere, but philosophically I wanted to climb a building. Why? They don't compare to Mt. McKinley or Mount Everest by any means, but they are symbolic representations of the boredom syndrome in modern society. For five years I'd been confined within a building, working nine to five like so many other people, yet never feeling at ease, wishing all the while I were free of such constraints so I could explore the real me. Yes, I was climbing a building like the animal climbing its cage from the outside, getting to the top, surmounting the territory so you know the cage can no longer hold you.

Analysis of Risk Factors   The fear of heights was critical in terms of managing the risks. It required a gradual desensitization to the point where I could relax and gain control of the fears. To accomplish this, I designed a ten-step program. At the start I merely stood as close as possible to the full window facings at lower floors and observed the wide expanse of the city. Slowly I moved to higher floors, practicing deep breathing while imagining myself climbing up the extrusions (rails) that run vertical to the building. These rails help guide the huge window-washing scaffold up and down during the twice-annual window cleanings. The final steps in this desensitization process involved actually riding up and down the outside of the building during one such cleaning. I made a total of six trips from top to bottom and back. To give you some idea how beautiful this transition from total fear to total control came about, I have included some descriptions from my journal.

On the morning of May 2nd, I climbed into the window washing rig. It was then that I experienced profound total body fear. I think the worst kind of death would be to fall from a great height, trying to blot out the reality of an impending impact, wanting to be snatched from the dreams jarring conclusion

. . . cranked out over the edge of the rooftop, hanging by guidewires 415 feet above the concrete pavement and swaying back and forth in the wind, my legs stiffened, my knees wobbled, and my knuckles turned white from my grip on the handrail. I ask myself a now familiar question, 'God, what am I doing here?' It's that feeling of being so quickly propelled outside your comfort zone, of projection into another dimension of awareness where your roots of security have been severed, that you find yourself psychologically isolated from any fixed reference point, groping for some familiar cue to interpret your feelings.

And yet, some six weeks later I noted in my journal:

By the third drop, I had made amazing progress. I could lean over the rail without my safety line, look down in relaxed fashion even while hanging at 415 feet. I frequently talked to myself, put positive tapes into the computer. I was gaining control. It felt so good inside to feel the accelerated changes taking place, coming to terms with such a fear. By the fourth drop I could even stand on the rail with no safety line and lean against the building like one of the window washers. By the sixth drop, I felt I'd mastered the fear. I even looked forward to going over the edge, for it had become a happy experience. Up high like that the air smells so clean and pure, and you can see all the points of interest around the city, all the elegant dining spots you've visited, and even the mighty Missouri winding itself between the forgotten back alleys of warehouses, grain storage elevators, and factories. How peaceful from this perch, watching the cars and trucks circulating through the city's veins of streets and major thoroughfares. It gave a feeling of supremacy, of mastery, like the pilot who, once airborne in a strange city, suddenly knows where everything is. Breaking through I call it. I'd finally broken through.

Another key factor was the equipment, building the proper device to assure my safety. The art and science of climbing buildings required a device that was fast, efficient, lightweight, and nondestructive to the building.

It was with great frustration and perseverance that the devices were finally built. Everyone was worried about liability in the event of some mishap. The devices were simple in their operation, consisting of spring-loaded cams that easily slid upward but locked in place when weight was applied in a downward direction. Teflon surfaces prevented scraping.

Back-Up Systems   By now you understand the value of this for managing risks (of *any* kind as we'll see later in the book). Just to give you some idea of this application to the climb, I had not one but *two* spring-loaded cams on each device. In addition, I had another caming device attached to my waist for extra safety. Also, I actually tested the devices on an exact replica of the building rail prior to the climb. But the best back-up system you can have is a second *and* third expert opinion. I consulted *three* separate engineers to confirm the effectiveness and safety of the climbing devices prior to the actual stunt. This third opinion has great implications in medicine, business, educational goals, as well as stunts.

Fitness and Nutrition As usual I ran for high energy and the tranquilizer effects it bestowed. But, given the specific demands of this experiment, I also did step-ups each day, 500 in ten minutes on a 20-inch bench while carrying a ten-pound pack. This represented a vertical distance of 800 feet, well beyond the actual climbing distance. To supplement this, I also trained with weights, working especially the forearms and triceps since the demands of climbing were greater there.

By now I had begun to ascertain certain basic principles regarding diet, which helped control fear, improve my general mood, and maximize my energy levels. I called it the Primitive Diet because of the high fiber content and absence of processed foods.

Visualization You *must* put the proper images in the psychic computer, begin to believe it has already happened. This is the formula, REALITY = Imagination × Vividness. Positive thoughts become your reality. Great achievers do this instinctively. To facilitate this process use photos whenever possible, but try to create the success scenario. Blown-up photos taken from the rooftop of the veterans memorial, Penn-Valley Park, Union Station, Crown Center Complex, and parking lots below helped me imagine myself doing the stunt. Even while stepping on my bench I'd look up, imagine the top and say to myself, "There it is, Mark; watch it come toward you."

Stress Management (Self Control) The forty-five minutes it took me to climb the building was the greatest happiness of my forty-year life. There are always problems you can't anticipate—when the devices stuck in the expansion gaps between floors; when the cams began to slip because perspiration streamed down my arms onto the rails. But *you do not panic!* You stop for a moment to observe the still nighttime city mirrored against the glass, to achieve the feel of belonging in that spot. You calmly resolve the problem. On you climb, moving the foot cam upward, then the waist cam, and on and on. A rhythm develops. You get lost in this rhythm, finally you're in flow, you perform each motion as though you'd been there many times before. You become the building, its atoms run through you and your nerve impulses through it. The building has being, and as you power up its vertical face you feel as safe as if gravity did not exist. That is happiness, coming to love what you once feared the most.

After reaching the top I pondered in my journal the risks I had taken:

> I turned to watch the caravan of cars, bumper to bumper headed downtown on the trafficway. How many overweight people, racing the clock, headed for boring jobs, maybe even smoking? I can't get life insurance but they can. Yet I am healthier than ever before. So who manages risk and who doesn't?

Epilogue In the cool fall of an evening when the bright orange maple leaves still flutter onto the courtyard below the building, you may find me there reflecting upon it all. The aura of the building is gone, though I remember well standing down here unable to see it happening, look up and be chilled in my own fear. But now it has, and I'm a better risk taker.

The vice president of the insurance company that owned the building invited me to his country club for dinner. He asked a hundred questions; I helped relieve his boredom. Oh well, the red snapper was superb.

Wellness Experiments

For a mentally handicapped child to run 100 yards, or a normal child to ride a horse, for an older person to try roller skating, or a claustrophobic to ride an elevator, the risks may seem as great as the experiments I've described. Risk taking is relative to each person's skill, perception of fear, and need system. Nevertheless, in each case wellness requires the same approach to ensure a safe and fun adventure.

Though my risky ventures seemed varied, *all* contained many wellness components. Foremost was the need to analyze the risk factors: the environmental aspects, the need for training (experience), and the use of proper equipment are all variables that determine the personal safety quotient. Once so identified, a plan of action is formulated to control the variables.

Second was the notion of back-up systems—having an alternative action plan if something goes wrong. Anticipate what *could* go wrong. This isn't negative thinking. It's foresight.

Third was the need to manage stress, to stay in control by relaxing, visualizing goals, being sensitive to the environment and people in that environment, enjoying the present, being patient and remaining calm in a crisis, and pursuing one's own uniqueness.

Fitness and nutrition provide the energy and strength to keep you in control and give you confidence that things will go as planned or, at the very least, that you can handle the unforeseen.

I knew about these wellness components before I experimented with extreme risk to resolve my boredom. But now I know my life, casual as it was, was more in danger then.

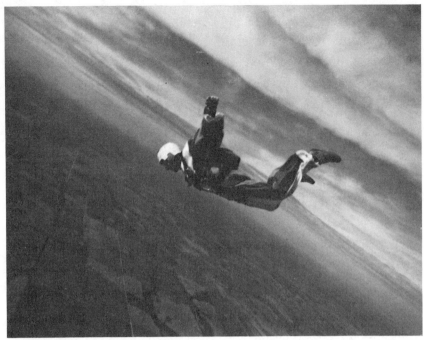

Skydiving is a confrontation with the unknown. But the risks are so intensified, they force you to be prepared, unlike the risks of a mundane lifestyle.

CHAPTER 3
Selected References

Fiske, Donald, and Salvatore R. Maddi. *Effects of Monotonous and Restricted Stimulation,* Chapter 5 from Functions of Varied Experience. Homewood, Ill: Dorsey Press, Inc., 1961.

Goldberger, Leo and R. Holt. *Experimental Interference with Reality Contact: Individual Differences,* Chapter 9 from Sensory Deprivation. P. Solomon, et al (ed.), Cambridge, Mass: Harvard University Press, 1961.

Risk Taking Is Stress Management

When you risk for wellness, it means giving up those behaviors that are familiar, comfortable, secure, and maybe even "normal." When I began running twenty years ago, a lot of my friends called me crazy and joked about my longevity ("We'll read about you getting run over by a Mack truck next year, Crookse.") Well, no Mack trucks have hit me yet, and those hecklers look about ten to fifteen years older than I do now. And, of course, now that it's "fashionable" to be seen running, they're doing it too.

As the wellness model in Section I portrays, high-level wellness means you take responsibility for your own health destiny. It means you embrace those wellness skills and challenges that can lead to new growth, higher energy levels, and peak performance. In order to do this, you need to grasp one simple, yet seldom recognized, truth:

> Stress is absolutely necessary for achieving high levels of performance in any field. It's the way we achieve our optimal level of stimulation, thus defeating Public Enemy Number One, boredom.

The athlete under the stress of competition exemplifies this notion. Under such conditions, not during practice, world records are set. But winning athletes prepare themselves mentally and physically, using wellness skills to make stress work for them.

For most of us, however, the "technological shock syndrome" has left few environmental opportunities to fulfill this need in modern life.

> The supermarket aisle has replaced the hunt, the automobile has replaced exploration by foot, and the secondhand has replaced the movement of a shadow across the Earth.

So, we have to create challenges, create the demands and stresses that can propel us to new growth. Failure to develop wellness skills leads to "dis-stress" (and eventually *dis-ease),* a feeling that you are out of control. Madison Avenue knows you are bored, and plays upon your needs for excitement and stimulation. Bad habits develop because they offer a temporary gratification, you get more lethargic and bored, and the vicious cycle continues.

This section will help you break that cycle. It will offer positive forms of stimulation such as learning to enjoy the crunch of food to explore the diversity of fitness, to make movies with your mind, communicate better, and even explore your body's responses while in a weightless environment. So, let's be risk takers. Leave that comfort zone behind and soar to new heights.

CHAPTER 4

Visualization: Find Your Own Cave

Where there is no vision the people perish.
—Proverbs 29:18

A Backward Glance

Even cave dwellers understood the importance of positive thinking. They *had* to be positive when survival required hunting prey, as large as the 1,500-pound cave bear.

The hunters achieved this by visualizing the event beforehand, creating all the detailed vividness necessary to program the mind with positive thoughts. They would then perform certain religious or magical rituals before the hunt to strengthen the power of this wish picture.

This is not merely conjecture. The evidence of cave paintings strongly supports it. First, large numbers of animals were painted with spears in them, in many cases with blood spewing from the nose and mouth. Second, there was the peculiar practice of superimposing one painting on another, suggesting that a new picture was made not so much for display as for new magic, for a future hunt and a different animal. Finally, much of this art appears not in open cave homes with easy access to the outside, but in deep, uninhabitable, subterranean caves. They served not as homes, but as shrines, and the art was not intended to give pleasure to the beholder. Its sole purpose was to give the hunter more of a feeling of control over the hunt by implanting positive images in his mind. He would focus upon these images, often while engaged in religious rituals.

The Current Situation

Many of us have, amid the fast pace of modern living, forgotten how to use our minds to the fullest. We need to be childlike once again. As

40

children we were naturally expressive, for children always think in pictures and their little minds are full of imaginings and wild possibilities. Left to themselves, they will make an adventure of life from the barest of raw materials. How else could a deck of cards become a house or a milk carton become a boat?

But confronted by the reality principle, that dreams require effort, many of us stop visualizing. This is unfortunate because it is only by maintaining these images that thoughts get translated into action. Part of the problem is that we don't use this technique to the fullest. In fact, neurophysiologists say we only use 6 to 10 percent of our brain capacity.

The right hemisphere is the portion of the brain designed for creating images and for projecting thought patterns of desired goals, outcomes, and actions into other areas of the brain. Now more than ever before we need to revive this childlike quality in order to overcome any obstacles that stand between us and our aspirations. We can achieve great things. The tool resides in all of us. Let's learn how to better use this technique.

Visualization means constructing a mental image of yourself success-fully completing some goal. It can be something achieved readily or in the distant future. The technique is basically the same, except the farther removed in time the goal is the *more* you will need to use and refine the mental images. This is because there will be more obstacles. We live in a crowded, competitive society and only by using these techniques often and correctly can you program the subconcious (the computer) to respond to your thought pictures (input) with appropriate action (output).

In one dramatic example, members of the Swiss Alpine skiing team were taught the skills of visualization and its counterpart, mental rehearsal. After they had practiced these skills for awhile, the skiers were sent down the grand slalom course, backpacks filled with equipment to monitor brain waves, heart rate, and muscle tension. The next day in the laboratory, the skiers again hooked up to the monitors and were asked to imagine them-selves running the slalom. The physiologic responses (much easier to measure than mental or emotional ones) were exactly the same, whether they were actually skiing well or only imagining it.

In another study, two groups of twenty boys were matched for their ability to shoot free throws: at the start of the study, both groups were equal in overall performance. One group actually practiced 30 minutes per day every day, shooting free throws, for one whole month. During this same month, the other group of twenty boys practiced *mentally,* also for 30 minutes. Guess what happened? When they brought both groups back at the end of the 30-day test period, *both* groups had improved significantly in their ability to make free throws. But, here is the amazing result. There was *no difference* in the two groups' performance, whether they practiced mentally or actually shot free throws!

We can draw two conclusions:

1. You can try things out mentally before you actually do them and explore the options.
2. Once you do them you can improve much faster by rehearsing or practicing mentally as well as physically.

However, the best results will occur when both techniques are being used. By doing both the work and the mental rehearsal, you give yourself the best of all possible chances to become a winner. Remember how our primitive ancestors painted their goal to have a better image of it? Recall that this technique was used in virtually every one of the feats. While preparing for the 91-foot-bridge jump, I not only practiced by doing progressively higher jumps to perfect my skills, I also used photo overlays and positive imagery to prepare mentally. Both were important. To have used only mental images or visualization may not have been sufficient, given the dramatic, high-risk nature of that jump. Perhaps a 30- or 40-foot jump would have been quite achievable using visualization techniques alone.

During the trip down the Missouri River, there were times when I could not visualize myself completing the swim/float. At those times I changed the goal such as images or pictures in my brain to a more achievable goal such as just getting around the next bend, or just getting to the next city. The important point was that *I always kept using the technique,* even though I had to refine and modify the images that went into my brain. We must continue to maintain some image that represents a step forward toward our goal and this image should therefore be a positive one. *At no time* did I ever see myself sick or allow other negative images to enter my mind. This is very important.

During my 9,000-foot first-time freefall from an airplane, my death concerns were enormous. I had to fight constantly to imagine freefalling in the jumper's arch correctly.

I even used a trampoline to help give me some idea of what to expect so I could incorporate this into my mental picture. As it turned out, a minor malfunction did occur, the result of my falling so stably the air current could not open my pilot chute.

The use of visualization was also described in my preparation for the building climb. Remember how I practiced step-ups with a rail in front of me similar to the actual rail on the building? Remember how I described the intricate details I imagined in my mind as though I was actually climbing?

Earl Nightingale, noted author and speaker, says, "Whatever it is that you would like to do better, act as though you are a top-flight expert at it. If you continue to play this part long enough, you will become an expert." He cites the example of Arnold Palmer, who at ten years old was on his way to becoming the world's greatest golfer. He used to pretend that he was playing in national tournaments. He would then attempt to be the sports commentator announcing that the champion, Arnold Palmer, was now getting ready to tee off.

If you can create a mental image of the person you would most like to become, begin now to act as that person would act in everything that you do. Gradually, imperceptibly, you will become that person. The whole secret is to use the visualization technique, to hold fast in your mind the mental image of the person you would most like to be. Then, in every situation, act and talk as you feel that the person would.

Muhammad Ali, in his book, *The Greatest,* provides a stirring description of how visualization helped transform him into the world champion he later became.

> I start dreaming. I can see myself telling my next door neighbor, "I'm getting ready to fight for the Heavyweight Title of the World!", and coming back next night to say, "I'm now the Heavyweight Champion of the World!!". I start watching a fight on TV with more interest. What catches my eye is the way fighters trade punches with each other. I see Ralph "Tiger" Jones, Hurricane Jackson, Carmen Basilio, Gene Fullmer, and watch how they stand, and get hit with the same punch, or jab each other over and over. And I know I can beat them. Even when I see Archie Moore, I know that one day I will be able to whip these men very easily, because they are not moving, not circling, not moving backwards at the right time. I know I can learn to hit without getting hit. I can see it.

Even his poetic phrase, "Float like a butterfly, sting like a bee," represents positive imagery (visualization). In picturing such images he imagines himself dancing lightly, easily, conserving energy and quickly striking his opponent when he sees an opening.

Other well-known athletes professing to use this technique include Dave Parker of the Pittsburgh Pirates; Mark Fydrich, Detroit Tigers; Drew Pearson, Dallas Cowboys, Renaldo Nehemiah, World Record Holder, 110-meter hurdles. Said Jean-Claude Killy, "you don't need snow to improve your skiing. Just think of your mind as a computer and start erasing those old tapes. Re-program yourself."

Visualization is currently being used in a wide variety of ways in many fields. Almost all artists, whether in art, music, or drama learn to become very proficient at this technique, since creativity, by its very nature, requires that we first develop a mental image of what it is we wish to produce. In the health field, visualization is being used to help people give up bad habits like smoking and drinking excessively. It's also used to promote relaxation.

Visualization is being used in holistic medicine and natural healing to control or cure disorders ranging from high blood pressure to cancer, our dread disease. For example, since 1965, Dr. Carl Simonton of Fort Worth Texas, a radiologist specializing in cancer treatment, has been successfully treating cancer patients with this technique. Normally, most patients who visit his center are diagnosed as having terminal cancer, that is, the cancer is considered so advanced that no conventional cure is deemed possible. Using his techniques, 60 percent of 152 patients reported in one study showed relief of symptoms and an improvement of their general condition. Those patients who failed to show such improvement also demonstrated poor cooperation in applying the visualization techniques. It is not uncommon to see tumors gradually shrinking in size on X-ray. I had the opportunity to see serial brain scans taken from a 14-year-old boy after treatment with this technique at the Menninger Clinic in Topeka, Kansas. The tumor gradually shrunk until it was no longer visible on a brain scan. The examining surgeons could not believe how the "terminal" patient recovered with no trace of the cancerous tumor.

As Dr. Simonton soon discovered, visualization and its successful use depend, more than anything else, upon individualizing the type of images to fit each person's expectations. For example, one person may be able to relax successfully by visualizing a quiet, peaceful, mountain scene. Another would relax better with images of large ocean waves crashing against rocks. One wonderful advantage of visualization is that each person can "try on" several different images and see how he or she responds to each one. For example, you may wish to ask for a raise from your employer by visualizing several alternatives to accomplish this objective. In fact, you could also role play the situation by acting out each of these imagined situations. Also, visualize several possible reactions from your boss and imagine your counter-responses to each possible reaction. In this way, by rehearsing beforehand, you can be better prepared to handle all the possible outcomes.

Art Linkletter, once told about how Walt Disney took him to a spot one day and described in intricate detail his dream of Disneyland. Art Linkletter couldn't share the same images. He failed to invest $5,000 that would have made many millions for him.

The TV show "That's Incredible" featured an architect who was blind and yet could design houses in his mind down to the last minute detail. This demonstrates how effective the technique can be, once mastered.

In each of the feats previously described, I used my fear constructively by imagining all of the possible negative outcomes and then preparing myself to deal with each contingency.

This further ensured my safety and helped me achieve my goal.

I have already mentioned some of the uses of visualization to help you understand what a potent tool it can become if used regularly. Let me now briefly list all its current applications in health and wellness in case you choose to improve yourself in one of these areas after mastering the technique.

Uses of Visualization in Wellness

Enhancement of Self-image   Use it to eliminate unwanted behavior patterns, attitudes, and habits. This increases self-esteem and builds a positive mental attitude. Imagine yourself as an important person who has much to offer other people. Imagine yourself being assertive, letting others know your needs and seeing them respect you for this openness.

Enhancement of Sports Performance This has already been mentioned and is one of the areas currently being widely explored among college and professional sports teams. Concentration and guided imagery can implant success pictures in the athlete's mind. The average middle-aged woman might try to imagine herself fit and see herself participating in various aerobic sports. This will enhance motivation to follow through in actual participation.

Weight Control Being overweight is a symptom, not a cause; visualization can be used to imagine yourself slim. Imagine eating only the right foods independent of emotional factors which trigger poor eating habits. Imagine how great you look in the mirror with the body you can have.

Smoking Cessation Since much evidence cites smoking as a stress-reduction technique, by learning to relax properly and imagine yourself as a healthy nonsmoker you can replace the dependence on this substance. Imagine yourself being offended by the very smell of smoke, by dirty ashes, and smoky places.

Stress Symptom Reduction Tension headaches, upset stomach, low back pain, and high blood pressure can be reduced by focusing on specific areas of your body and imagining the particular area functioning in a healthy way. For example, imagining your blood vessels dilate may lower blood pressure and headaches and imagining muscles as elongated rubber bands that gradually let go may reduce some common stress symptoms.

Recovery from Illness or Injury All you need do is focus upon what constitutes the healing or recuperative process and continue to see this process taking place. Imagine a wound healing by seeing in your mind the healthy tissue growing back and new supplies (nutrients) coming into the wound.

Better Sleep Project each day as happy, relaxing, and frustration free. Put yourself in a restful frame of mind. Then stand back and see yourself sleeping soundly like a baby. Hear yourself breathing calmly and deeply and imagine having beautiful dreams of carefree experiences.

Overcoming Fears Fear is the greatest obstacle to human progress. Some experience it as vague anxiety, others as an imagined outcome. Through visualization you can imagine yourself performing various activities of a fearful nature, which you could not yet do in reality. Imagine yourself speaking to an audience, expressing your deeper feelings to someone, or confronting a co-worker about some issue. Be vivid in your imagination and practice it until you begin to believe it has happened. This gives the confidence to finally confront the fear situation.

Goal Achievement *Anything* you want can be visualized and ultimately achieved if you believe it deep enough. Break the goal down into much smaller components and visualize each and every small component while still retaining the overall picture of the final result.

Learning the Procedure

Now is the time to get down to the actual basics of learning to use these techniques. First, understand what it is you want to accomplish and then proceed through the steps as outlined. First, let's see to what degree you are already using the technique. You may be using it but not fully harnessing it to your full advantage.

Visualization Quiz

1. Do you consciously daydream or focus attention on events to come?   Yes   No

2. Are most of the images in these daydreams positive in nature?   Yes   No

3. Are your images vivid (detailed) as opposed to vague?   Yes   No

4. Do you allow at least ten continuous minutes of each mental imagery?   Yes   No

5. Do you use techniques for a wide variety of problem areas (success in sports, creative pursuits, business goals, etc.)?   Yes   No

6. When imagining certain situations and or outcomes, do you utilize other sensory modalities such as smell, feel, and sound as well as the visual, do you see in colors?   Yes   No

7. D you combine visualization with various types of music in order to release the right brain (creative side) for assisting in strengthening such images?   Yes   No

8. Do you use visual images to relax (beach scenes, etc.)   Yes   No

9. Do you keep modifying your "movie" according to new information or input gained from actual practice?   Yes   No

10. Do you take or use photographs to sharpen your focus when using this technique?   Yes   No

SCORING: Give yourself one point for each Ys-18es. A score of 9-10 is excellent; 7-8, good; 5-6, fair; and 0-4, poor.

If you scored at least 6 in the Yes column, you are already using visualization in a productive way. You just need to refine it and make a more conscious effort to build it into your mind on a regular basis. Perhaps just making an effort to score 8 to 10 will serve as your goal once the basic technique is explained.

1. Select an area in which you wish to improve yourself. Be general at first. Examples: Health, communication and self-expression.
2. Relax your body. Try to free your mind from other distractions, that is, the little, everyday trivia. Get in a comfortable position,

perhaps in a dark room. Then breathe slowly and deeply. Keep your jaw loose and relaxed.

3. Begin to see the fine details of what you want to achieve. Concentrate on them. You are the director, producer, and camera operator in this movie sequence. Change the details or the action in any way that you wish.

4. Sense the feelings associated with your goal. Let your mind and body experience them.

5. Now let your other senses experience them. What are the smells, the sounds, and the physical sensations?

6. Silently or speaking aloud, tell yourself in so many words that you deserve to achieve the goals you are imagining.

7. Still breathing deeply, trust and believe that you will have the success that you see, hear, and feel in this mental movie. Positive thinking does have power, if you put your will and energy behind it.

8. If you have difficulty concentrating do this: Find pictures (or take photos) or have someone talented in art draw your "wish picture" to increase the vividness of the image. Remember, Reality = Imagination x Vividness. For example, having an actual artistic drawing (or photo) of yourself at a lighter weight will help you program the computer. Carry these actual pictures with you and keep them in your thoughts.

9. Practice, practice, practice. Become a better artist in defining your image. Make this a daily routine. Remember, modern living often robs us of our dreamtime. I will conclude this chapter with four exercises in visualization. Please try them.

Visualization Exercises

Exercise 1.   Sensory Integration.
Purpose: Awareness of mind-body connection. Relax as previously described. Breathe deeply with eyes closed.
Image: A lemon, a knife, a cutting board.
Activity: Cutting lemon into 6 slices
Observation: Smell, color of pulp, sound of knife against skin of lemon and on cutting board.
Activity: Squeeze lemon slice on tongue.
Reactions: Expressions, feelings, and sensations.

Exercise 2.   Problem Solving.
Purpose: Explore possible options. Relax again. Breathing deeply is always important.
Decision: How to spend my time this weekend?
Images: Movie theatre, exercising in some way, concert, travel some-

place, museum, sporting event, working, dining out. Cut pictures from magazines to help you get some good images if necessary.

Activity: Whichever ones you choose to imagine; go through each one and imagine different companions if this is a question, different locations, different outcomes. Use as many senses as possible.

Reactions: Feelings from each activity or person. Which one was the most satisfying?

Exercise 3.   Goal Setting.

Purpose: Self satisfaction.

Decision: What things in life are important to me?

Images: Picture very specifically images of yourself accomplishing something you desire to achieve, a vacation you wish to pursue, or other desired achievements. Remember, this goal can be in any area of your life: health, sports, finance, love, etc. See in three dimensions. Incorporate lots of motion.

Activity: After you have imagined what behaviors are necessary to a person who would accomplish this goal, visualize yourself doing these things. Remember, "When the person and the goal become equated, the goal must be satisfied." This means when the images become vivid enough in your mind from regular practice, you will seek out people, places, and actions consistent with reaching that goal.

Observation: Successful lovers, businessmen, artists, sports figures, etc. What characteristics do they possess? Imagine *you* also possess these qualities. Be as vivid as possible in constructing your mental motion-picture scenery.

Reactions: How did it feel to accomplish your goal? How did others react to you?

Exercise 4.   Weight loss.

Purpose: Wellness enhancement. Remember to relax in a place where you will not be disturbed.

Decision: How to best lose weight so it will stay off permanently?

Images: With eyes closed, pretend you are someone else standing off to the side looking at your body. You have a special pair of magic glasses. Everytime you blink, the outline of your subject *(you!)* will begin to shrink, especially in the areas of high fat deposition. See yourself getting thinner. Use this shrinking image several times daily, especially when hungry. See yourself walking in a nice setting. See yourself eating low-fat foods. See how positively your friends respond to you, how excited old friends act as you actually *do* shrink. See how good you look in a new, fashionable outfit. Imagine how much more people will want to touch you, hug you, be around you because your confidence is growing and you exude joy.

Activity: Think up all the sports or activities you can do to keep busy, especially before eating. Imagine the fun you will have getting outdoors more often in the sunlight and fresh air.

Observation: Women who have successfully lost weight. How do they act? Talk to them and listen to their satisfaction, their enthusiasm. Imagine yourself becoming this enthused. Observe thin people having fun, touching, laughing. Imagine all these things happening to you as you shrink in size.

Reactions: How does it feel to see yourself thinner? How does it feel to be proud of the thin body you imagine? How does it feel to be able to look at fattening foods and not be tempted?

Once you master this technique, you should be able to answer "rarely" to a great many questions in the *Life Risk Questionnaire* in Chapter 1. By using positive mental imagery you will not only become mentally stronger, you will be better equipped to make wise decisions regarding risks in your everyday life. Some of your daily sources of distress should decrease or disappear.

CHAPTER 4
Selected References

Samuels, Mike, and Nancy Samuels. *Seeing With the Mind's Eye— Techniques and Uses of Visualization.* Random House, 1979.

Simonton, Carl. *The Value of Positive Mental Images,* Chapter 12 from Getting Well Again. Tarcher Publishing Co., 1978.

CHAPTER 5

Exercise: Trade In Your Spear for Jogging Shoes

A Backward Glance

Primitive man had to be fit. His life depended on it. And nature prepared him well to handle the stresses he faced. The primary mechanism of this is adrenalin, a hormone that calls forth carbohydrates from storage in the liver and pours them into the bloodstream in the form of sugar for immediate energy. This potent hormone also increases blood flow to the heart, lungs, central nervous system and limbs, while decreasing flow to the abdominal organs. Let me now recount an anthropologist's description of a typical day's hunt.

> The anticipation of the chase, the excitement of seeing and stalking an animal trigger off the adrenal response that will be needed to attack and kill it in a sudden burst of exertion. But this is only part of the activity. They often must follow an animal's spoor for many weary miles before coming upon it. Then tired as they may be, they must still summon the energy to sprint forward in hopes of planting a poisoned dart or spear before the animal runs out of range. If it is a large animal they may have to follow it doggedly for many miles, sometimes even days before they can close in and kill it. During this protracted chase they may eat only a handful of food to sustain them as they run.
>
> (Clark F. Howell, *Early Man,* Time-Life Books: 1970, pp. 172-73).

The Current Situation

Consider the modern plight. The businessman has been working diligently on an important proposal, one that could elevate him to a higher position in the company. But others within the company will oppose his ideas. There promises to be a war of viewpoints. He will have to aggressively defeat the arguments of others. He has been growing steadily more aroused and tense for the previous three days in anticipation of the board meeting. His system has been churning out adrenalin and when, during the actual confrontation, several people severly challenge his ideas, his blood sugar, cholesterol and fatty acids skyrocket. The meeting is adjourned until several days later. He needs a release. He finds a restaurant where he downs several cocktails, followed by a high-fat meal.

His adrenal gland cannot be blamed. It responded loyally as it has for thousands of years to a perceived danger. But the safety valve is now gone. There was no physical outlet to siphon off the buildup of hormones and other potentially dangerous substances. This was poor risk taking; the continued distress of such meetings can kill this person if the same pattern continues.

Being physically active and keeping fit is still the best way to handle this dilemma. A twelve-minute jog could have served as a defusing device, dispelling the adrenalin and other substances that were released. My own experiences with fear and the tranquilizer effect of exercise certainly taught me this.

I believe my ability to handle the emotional stress of jumping from an airplane may be attributed to my high fitness level. An EKG taken during the entire one-and-a-half-mile freefall showed a heart rate of only 152 beats/minute. Similar data on Air Force recruits has shown heart rates of 180-220 beats/minute. An experienced skydiver (more than 1,000 jumps) my own age had a heart rate of 148 beats/minute. He was overweight, smoked, and was in poor physical condition. Yet our stress response was almost identical, despite his greater experience.

I also firmly believe that being in peak physical condition helped me survive the 375 bitterly cold miles from Kansas City to St. Louis in the Missouri River. For nearly one week, I swam and floated some twenty hours per day, while expending about 8,000 calories per day. Climbing the building put great stress upon me mentally and physically. My weight training on the Nautilus machines played a major role in that successful enterprise. I was so keyed up, I ran four miles upon returning home.

Understanding Stress

Life is stress. We cannot (and should not) live without it. Show me someone with no stress and I'll show you a corpse. All living creatures have stress because everytime the heart beats, pressure is exerted on the wall of every little blood vessel in the body. Even when we're lying down our bodies are exposed to the stress of gravity, the pressure is being exerted upon the bones and their joint structures. It is not stress which is to be avoided, it's distress. *Distress* is a feeling of discomfort produced because we're not fully in control of the events taking place in our lives. Wellness (optimal health), achieved with proper exercise and good nutrition, can help us enormously in handling stress by increasing our stress tolerance limits.

This does not mean success in life cannot be achieved without guarding one's health; there are too many examples to the contrary. But, remember the admonition, "You spend your health to get your wealth, and then you spend your wealth to get it back again!" Certainly success may be achieved at the expense on one's health but you may not be around very long to enjoy it. Howard Hughes certainly amassed a great fortune but suffered a massive heart attack in his mid-fifties, preventing him from enjoying his fortune for a full lifetime. Elvis Presley, a multimillionaire, died at age forty-four, the result of a drug overdose. Both were poor risk takers.

Dr. Charles Garfield, a psychology professor at the University of California at San Francisco, has been studying high performers for fifteen years—people who turned out smarter, more capable, more successful than anyone might have predicted. In his research, Dr. Garfield found that high performers are healthier than average people and for hardheaded reasons. They know that when they are physically tired or wilting under mental stress, they are less efficient. So, they are never "too busy" for relaxation and exercise.

The question arises: "How does staying healthy and fit help people perform better and therfore increase their satisfaction?" It does this in a number of ways. It saves time (contrary to public opinion), helps us handle job stresses better, and also helps us think clearer and be more decisive in our judgments. Research studies at Boston State Hospital's Sleep Laboratory and at the University of Chicago indicate that

> those who sleep less than six hours a night are likely to be smooth and efficient, extroverted, decisive, ambitious, and self-confident, whereas those who required nine hours or more tended to be rebellious, opinionated, critical, chronic worriers, insecure, anxious, and indecisive.

Studies indicate physically fit people require less sleep, because their sleep is of better quality. What this means is that there's more extra time per week for the fit person to invest in other activities. They store more energy (glucose) in their muscles so they can accomplish more without experiencing fatigue. Physically fit people *look* for challenges. Therefore, they rarely experience boredom.

The Two Primary Patterns of Stress

Perhaps the best contribution physical fitness can provide is to improve stress tolerance, which is important if we are striving for a high, difficult-to-achieve goal. In wellness medicine we call it *peak performance*. Dr. Kenneth Pelletier, author of *Mind is Healer, Mind is Slayer,* and nationally recognized stress expert from the University of California at Berkeley,

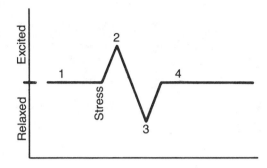

says there are two primary forms of stress, *short term* and *long term*. An example of the short-term type would be to have your car fail to start when you are already late for an appointment. You get out of the car, lift the hood, adjust the battery cable (which is slightly loose) and the car starts right up. You experience a feeling of relief. If your blood pressure were being monitored on a machine, a graph like the above would occur.

Point 1 is your baseline level before the stress. Point 2 is this stress reaction that involves increases in heart rate, blood pressure, blood sugar, and muscle tension. It corresponds to the firing of the sympathetic nervous system. Point 3, the period of compensatory relaxation after the stress has passed, corresponds to the firing of the parasympathetic nervous system. Point 4 is the return to the baseline. *This is the normal, healthy way of reacting to stress.* This kind of reaction occurred quite often in the two weeks prior to one of the stunts described earlier. During the course of the day, I'd build up tension thinking about the event. I would measure my blood pressure only to find it elevated at 150/84 mm. Hg. Then I'd go run four to five miles. Ten minutes later, the blood pressure was back to normal at 116/76 mm. Hg. The running served as a release; it dispelled the effects produced by the stress of the impending event. This is exactly what Dr. Herbert DeVries of USC found in his research on stress. He found that 30 minutes of brisk walking was a very potent tranquilizer in reducing muscle tension in a sample of older women. In fact, it proved more potent than a well-known tranquilizer drug (Meprobate). Also, the tranquilizer effect of the exercise was much longer in duration than that of the drug.

How about depression? Research evidence has shown that exercise, especially aerobic exercise, beats the blues. In 1976, University of Wisconsin psychiatrist Dr. John Griest found that regular jogging worked better than psychotherapy in overcoming moderate depression. Recent studies by Dr. Elizabeth Doyne at the University of Rochester indicate

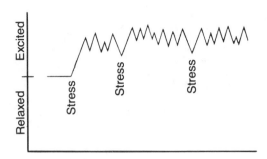

this antidepressant effect can begin in as short a time as five minutes after exercise begins.

Long-term stress is the type that really causes the trouble. Examples are job stress, family stress, emotional conflicts, and money difficulties, all the vague but ever-present problems and worries. They are what Dr. George Sheehan calls "the full court press of life." There seems to be no clear end point, no clear resolution to that kind of stress. I often tell people the feats were really *not that stressful.* Sure, they were intense in nature, but still they were relatively short lived. The other life stresses I had to deal with on a frequent basis, like financial worries, frequent delays in my plans, and worrying about how others might perceive me, were much much harder to deal with. Sometimes, during a confrontation with some-one I'll often think, "Phew, I'd rather climb a dozen buildings than go through this again." Buildings and other inanimate structures can be easily planned for and the risks controlled. You can't always predict how some-one might react or how they'll feel about something you did or said. There often seems to be no end, no clear resolution to that kind of stress. As I've already explained, all the bodily functions accelerate as though your life were in danger, and they stay elevated without release. We experience it as anxiety, frustration, tension, and worry. If we were to hook up someone in this kind of situation to a monitor, we'd see the graph that's illustrated above.

There is a level of high excitation without the compensatory relaxation phase. It's this kind of biological stress pattern that leads to disease. Cancer and heart disease are nonexistent in primitive countries of the world and social anthropologists believe the lack of social stress is one explanation for this.

Heart disease is our number one killer in the United States. In 1981, coronary heart disease killed more than one million Americans. Of the 1,200 cardiac deaths a day, almost half (43 percent) occurred on a Monday, strongly suggesting that distress, probably similar to that described, was a significant contributor in a great percentage of these deaths. According to one government study, three-fourths of all visits to family doctors and internists were related to distress with no apparent end point.

We need a way to calm down, to induce the relaxation or release phase. Aerobic exercise seems to do exactly this. Examples of aerobic activities are jogging, brisk walking, swimming, cycling, rowing, cross-country skiing, roller skating, and racketball. Sports like tennis and golf are normally too intermittent to provide the stimulation necessary for the heart and lungs to process oxygen for long durations. Aerobic activities utilize large muscle groups, actively contracting and relaxing in rhythmical fashion, thus promoting good overall body tone and an efficient circulatory system.

In recent years a great deal of research has focused upon such occupations as police, firefighters, and air traffic controllers. It is of interest to compare these occupations because of the different stresses each must confront. Firefighters and police spend a lot of time sitting or otherwise being sedentary. Then, when called into action, they are required to deal with the sudden intense type of stress. Firefighters, for example, may be required to go all out, performing activities like climbing, chopping, and pulling heavy equipment while wearing 50 to 60 pounds of clothing in a very hot, smoky environment. Heart rates of 160 to 190 beats/minute have been recorded on firefighters working up to two hours nonstop while subduing a fire. That's why it's so important they be physically fit. Police officers, many of whom smoke and sit in offices or patrol cars, may suddenly be required to pursue an offender on foot or in a high-speed chase. Many firefighters report poor sleeping habits while on duty at the fire station because they know they may be suddenly awakened. Studies conducted at UCLA and elsewhere have convincingly demonstrated that the incidence of injuries and stress-related disorders drops significantly after a well-rounded physical conditioning program of aerobic exercises, strength training, and flexibility exercises. Chief Hinson of the Macon, Georgia, fire department not only found that the number of firefighters treated for heat exhaustion decreased dramatically but even found that percentage of fire loss of buildings went down after the program was in full swing. Policemen's heart rates while on stakeout (sitting in a patrol car) have shown 150 beats/minute.

Air traffic controllers, because of the constant vigilance required to guide as many as twelve planes simultaneously to and from an airport, usually experience the second type of stress, the kind that offers no release. This results in distress and, ultimately, poor health. Ideally, they should be taught to relax periodically during the day or after work using meditation, exercise, or some form of visualization. This is rarely the case. Instead, according to psychiatrist Dr. Elliot Beneyra, who has treated many of these controllers, in an effort to rest his mind, the controller compounds the problem by drinking. If this routine continues week after week, the controller begins exhibiting the same symptoms we find in battle fatigue.

These people need aerobic exercise, not alcohol. And to guarantee high motivation they should be given time off (on premises) to exercise. The money the companies would save on early retirements would more than pay for such a program, because the problem is chronic, and temporary drug-induced releases often backfire.

In one study, two-thirds of the controllers at the O'Hare Airport in Chicago (considered the busiest airport in the United States), had ulcers or showed ulcer symptoms. Researchers at Boston University studied 400 controllers on the job and found extreme fluctuations in blood pressure in one-third to one-half of the men studied, during both hectic and slow days.

In short, the better the shape you're in, the better you can handle stress, and the less likely you'll be to get stuck in this chronic stress pattern.

How does exercise do this? It does this in two ways. First, exercise tends to burn up the blood fat and blood sugar mobilized by stress and also dispels some of the adrenalin and epinephrine (stress hormones) that keep you in a state of alarm. Research has also shown that habitual exercise decreases the tendency of white cells (platelets) to stick together, thereby offering further protection against distress. Even stomach acidity, which can lead to ulcers, has been shown to decrease with exercise conditioning. Finally, just making the decision to take time out for exercise will create a psychological mind set that will help you react differently to your job, your office, your sense of achievement, your career. It's the SLOW DOWN sign that helps us regain our focus.

How Badly Do You Need Exercise?

Drs. Perry London and Charles Spielberger in their research on stress have prepared a Temper Test and a Job Stress Index. It would be a good idea at this point for you to take these tests and find out where you rank in these measures of stress.

Temper Test: Are You Stress-prone?

DIRECTIONS: A number of statements that people have used to describe themselves are given below. Read each statement and then circle the appropriate number to indicate how you generally feel. There are no right or wrong answers. Do not spend too much time on any one statement, but give the answer which seems to describe how you generally feel.

	Almost Never	Some-times	Often	Almost always
1. I am quick tempered.	1	2	3	4
2. I feel annoyed when I am not given recognition for doing good work.	1	2	3	4

	Almost Never	Some-times	Often	Almost always
3. I have a fiery temper.	1	2	3	4
4. I feel infuriated when I do a good job and get a poor evaluation.	1	2	3	4
5. I am a hotheaded person.	1	2	3	4
6. It makes me furious when I am criticized in front of others.	1	2	3	4
7. I get angry when I'm slowed down by others' mistakes.	1	2	3	4
8. I fly off the handle.	1	2	3	4
9. When I get mad, I say nasty things.	1	2	3	4
10. When I get frustrated, I feel like hitting someone.	1	2	3	4

SCORING: Add up your points (1-4) for each item. Your total score will be somewhere between 10 and 40. A man who scores 17, or a woman who scores 18, is just about average. If you score below 13, you're well down in the safe zone but perhaps unresponsive to situations that provoke others. A score above 20 means you may be a hothead—scoring higher than three-quarters of those tested.

Job Stress Index: Are You Hassled?

DIRECTIONS: This survey lists 10 job-related events that have been identified as stressful by employees working in different settings. Please read each item and circle the number that indicates the approximate number of times during the past month that you have been upset or bothered by each event.

Number of Occurrences During the Past Month

1. I have been bothered by fellow workers not doing their job.	0	1	2	3 +
2. I've had inadequate support from my supervisor.	0	1	2	3 +
3. I've had problems getting along with co-workers.	0	1	2	3 +
4. I've had trouble getting along with my supervisor.	0	1	2	3 +
5. I've felt pressed to make critical on-the-spot decisions.	0	1	2	3 +
6. I've been bothered by the fact that there are not enough people to handle the job.	0	1	2	3 +
7. I've felt a lack of participation in policy decisions.	0	1	2	3 +
8. I've been concerned about my inadequate salary.	0	1	2	3 +
9. I've been troubled by a lack of recognition for good work.	0	1	2	3 +
10. I've been frustrated by excessive paperwork.	0	1	2	3 +

SCORING: To determine how your stress compares with other workers, add up the points that you circled for each item (0-3 +). Your score will be between 0 and 30. People who score between 5 and 7 are about average in how often they experience job-related stress. If you score higher than 9, you may have cause for concern. At 4 or lower, you have a relatively nonstressful job.

If you scored higher than 20 on temper and higher than 9 on the job stress index, you've got a dangerous combination going. Double-digit stress means you had better find a suitable way to dispell your anger (exercise over the noon hour as many corporate employees do) or change jobs. As I will emphasize later, this is not the best alternative. Such ongoing job stress, unrelieved by relaxation, will erode your health over the years much more than cataclysmic accidents.

A number of stress researchers have concluded that the major cause of *dis*tress is the accumulation of life events and various changes with such high frequency that the body's adaptive energy is depleted. For example, they assign a numbering scale to any of 43 life events, which include things like marriage, divorce, death of a loved one, change to a new job, etc. They feel that whether the event is good or bad makes no difference. It is the total amount of life events which, they believe, requires more adjustment and adaptation.

When the score reaches 300, they say you're a candidate for an illness or a major disease. This buildup of major life events assumes that *all* people respond to *an event* in the same manner, which is a very bad assumption to make. People *do not* respond to events in a stereotyped manner, like a programmed robot.

Their past experiences, their frustration tolerance (which is highly related to their fitness level), and other factors will all create wide variation in stress reactivity. For example, Dr. Suzanne Kobasa, of the City University of New York found that when subjects were divided into healthy and unhealthy subjects, the amount of life change failed to predict illness and disease, even when it was well beyond 300 points. The unhealthy subjects *did* show a tendency to break down as life events accumulated. Dr. Kobasa concluded that the healthy and hardy personality views life changes such as the loss of a job as an opportunity rather than a tragedy. They see such events as positive and they "roll with the punches." The unhealthy person, on the other hand, tends to view it as a disaster and lets it create a psychological drain upon already depleted resources. Thus, he or she breaks down in some fashion or another. Kobasa's advice to buffer stress:

1. Commitment—To job, spouse, family, social institutions, wellness (optimal health), and personal values.
2. Control over one's life—A feeling that you control life. Being fit is a good way to regain this feeling of control.
3. Challenge—Seeing change and adversity as a challenge to be met and mastered. The fit person's greater energy reserves allow them to better adapt (and adopt) this attitude.

Remember, this is the hallmark of high-level wellness, turning a crisis into an opportunity. Unfit people seek security, for instinctively they know their adaptation energy is very limited.

Cost Savings in Business and Industry

Finally, the healthy person is going to be more efficient in their daily activities. Research by members of the Association for Fitness in Business indicate that fit employees miss fewer work days per year due to sickness, have much better morale on the job, are 5 to 10 percent more efficient in job tasks, and cost the company less money on health insurance claims per year.

In one large-scale study, insurance claims were reduced by 35 percent among companies offering fitness and other health education programs to their employees. Another 4-year study conducted by Dr. Ismail at Purdue University compared nonexercisers to exercisers in terms of medical costs. Results showed that the average yearly medical costs for the non-exercisers was $390.53 as compared to $166.41 for those who exercised regularly. Participants in an exercise program at Kennecott Copper experienced a 55 percent reduction in medical care costs. Medical costs for Canada Life Assurance employees were $28.50 less per exercising employee.

A study by James M. Burke, an editor of Chicago's Business Insurance magazine, revealed that companies that initiated more than four health or wellness efforts in 1982 reported total medical and health costs at 6.9 percent of total payroll. Companies that took no health initiatives paid 9.3 percent—nearly one and a half times more.

And finally, in a rare break with municipal conservatism, taxpayer's money is being used for wellness purposes in Napa, California. Municipal employees work out at one of three fitness facilities and attend free lectures on nutrition, etc. The initial expense of $40,000 has been recovered three times over in savings from worker's compensation.

During the run for the 1984 U.S. presidency an article titled, "Candidates are physically fit for the presidency," appeared in many newspapers. It gave the vital statistics for each one of the candidates, and stated they were all "very fit and healthy" because their blood pressures and blood cholesterols "were in the normal range." Unfortunately, the normal range in the United States is very undesirable. The real truth is they were all in moderate health at best. All had cholesterols way over 190 (a wellness norm) and two had high blood pressure by American Heart Association standards. The job of U.S. president requires optimal health, especially since the life expectancy for U.S. presidents is only 67 years of age.

People who exercise regularly also have an improved ability to make quick decisions. Gavriel Salvendi, an industrial engineer at Purdue University, found that physically fit people are 60 percent more adept at making complex decisions than sedentary individuals. This is probably due to an enhanced cerebral oxygen uptake (blood flow to the brain), as many research studies suggest.

Stress on the job has been monitored on employees at NASA. The results are intriguing. For example, monitoring one executive during his daily routine showed that climbing three flights of stairs raised his pulse to 120 beats/minute. But an argument with his secretary raised it to 160. Conferences could also shoot the heart rate way up, as the monitoring showed.

Yes, fitness and wellness is well worth the investment. Have your employer contact the Association for Fitness in Business for a reference list of self-help materials and guidelines.

How Much Exercise is Needed?

How much is enough? How do we know how much exercise is necessary to stressproof ourselves? The findings of two eminent scientists shed light on this question.

Dr. Kenneth Cooper, the "father of aerobics" and author of many books on the subject, says that running more than fifteen miles a week yields "diminishing returns." Speaking at the White House Symposium on Physical Fitness and Sports Medicine, he said that after observing more than 21,000 people over ten years, he had found that running eleven miles a week satisfied most of the requirements of a cardiovascular conditioning program and that running more than fifteen miles a week increased the incidence of stress-related injuries.

Fifteen miles per week of walking or three hours per week of any aerobic activity significantly raises the amount of HDL cholesterol. HDL cholesterol is good because it helps scavenge LDL, the bad form of cholesterol that laminates the interior of the vessel with fat, and carries it out the bowels. Still, I advocate you do more than this, for reasons I'll explain later.

Dr. Ralph Paffenbarger, Jr., Professor of Epidemiology at the Stanford School of Medicine, has studied over 17,000 subjects for almost twenty years. One of the first scientists to provide solid evidence that chronic exercise lengthens lifespan, he states, "The adjusted death rates of the most sedentary group were almost twice as high as those of the most active group."

Dr. Paffenbarger found that the ideal energy expenditure per week to reduce risk of heart disease amounted to 2,000 calories per week. For most people, this would be equal to about fifteen to eighteen miles of walking or jogging per week. To determine how many calories you burn for each mile you walk or jog, simply multiply your weight by 0.7.

Other activities will also do the job. Here's a list of calories burned per hour for various activities.

Activity	Calories Burned/hr
Swimming (freestyle)	800
Swimming (breaststroke)	500
Tennis (singles)	500
Tennis (doubles)	350
Golf (walking)	300
Racquetball	800
Skiing (downhill)	600
Skiing (cross-country)	550-700
Cycling (10 mph)	500
Roller skating	500
Stair-stepping (12-15 min.)	300

Additional Benefits of Exercise

There's another way vigorous exercise may stressproof you. It is called "jogging fever" and it doesn't mean enthusiasm. Ever stop to think about why your body temperature goes up when you have a systemic infection? It goes up to fight off the infection, since many foreign or bacterial agents are destroyed with even slight temperature elevations. Well, recent evidence now shows that during vigorous exercise, when the body temperature goes up three to four degrees above normal, harmful bacteria in the body may be destroyed. This practice bestows a sort of exercise-induced immunity against infectious agents.

Even when poor lifestyle habits and the effects of long term distress have resulted in heart disease, aerobic exercise may halt the disease progression. In one of the few well-controlled studies to determine this, Dr. Ronald Selvester, a cardiologist at Los Amigos Hospital in Downey, California, found that subjects who attained high fitness levels were able to halt the placquing process that eventually blocks blood flow and causes heart attack. Subjects who failed to improve their fitness levels did not show this effect and the disease continued to progress.

One recent study on people who exercise regularly has even shown that aerobic exercises like walking, cycling, etc. can decrease the probability of getting colon cancer. When you think about it, this makes a lot of sense. Such activities help speed the passage of food through the digestive system, decreasing the available time for carcinogens to form.

There is one other very little known (and little publicized) benefit of exercise. It decreases the rate at which the skin ages, because when you exercise vigorously, the tiny muscles that control the opening and closing of the pores get exercised and this helps maintain tonus of that organ. The skin is the largest organ of the body. Elimination of toxins through perspiration also takes a load off the liver, whose primary function is detoxification.

Exercise as Sensation Seeking

Since I am advocating that aerobic exercise can serve as a wellness challenge, then it should also provide enough stimulation to offset other more negative risks, like smoking, etc. Does it do this? The evidence, though scant, is very suggestive.

Dr. Carlos Perry, Director of Psychiatric Residency Training at the U.S. Air Force Medical Center in San Antonio, says,

> I think some chemical mediator is involved; some chain of biochemical events is caused by exercise. I agree with those who think sensory stimulation plays a role. The brain requires a certain amount of stimulation and if it doesn't get it, will try to provide that stimulation itself. So, if you have an inactive patient who shuts himself out from everything into a fantasy world, some form of kinesthetic stimulation (neuromuscular feedback to the brain) may be the only thing that can open him up to other forms of stimulation. Then you can break the cycle of sensory deprivation by restoring the needed sights, sounds, tastes, and smells.

Several studies on cigarette smoking and running suggest that as running mileage increases there is less tendency to smoke. One study found this to occur at about three miles per day. A survey on over a thousand participants of Atlanta's annual Peachtree Marathon found that over 80 percent had given up smoking after several months of running. Perhaps this is due to the stimulation of more oxygen to the brain. At any rate, aerobic (endurance) activities are certainly a great way to offset the boredom of modern life and beat the blahs. What about nonaerobic types of exercise?

There is a tendency for inactive people to misperceive the weight and boundaries of their bodies, to develop a distorted body image, especially as they grow older. As Dr. Raymond Harris points out in his book, *Guide to Fitness After Fifty,* the cure is movement, enough to generate more feedback (neuromuscular stimulation) to the brain. As Dr. Harris points out, "Muscular movements initiate stimuli in muscle spindles which are essential for optimal functioning of the central nervous system."

Muscle spindles, little biological amplifiers embedded in the muscles, relay information to the brain about muscle length, change of size, and rate of contraction. They are very responsive to changes in tension (resistance) placed upon the muscles, as in weightlifting. Weightlifting, body building, etc. all involve stimulation of these little amplifiers, which in turn increase stimulation and sensation. If done carefully, it can be a very satisfying experience.

In the normal course of soft living, we fail to stimulate our muscles enough. When we're suddenly required to lift a 50-pound bag of dog food, spare tire, or armload of firewood, we aren't conditioned for it. A severe strain or sprain may result.

Weight Lifting and Stress Control

Let's see now how our ancestors got by without barbells. Our Cro-Magnon ancestors of 20,000 years ago had very powerful physiques, as anthropologists gauge from analysis of their skeletal contours. The task of survival created its own weightlifting. For example, many seminomadic hunters who lived in the almost treeless landscape of Russia's Don River Valley would scavenge the bones and tusks of large mammoths. These often weighed up to 100 pounds. They might have to be carried for many miles since they were used for tools, weapons, and shelter.

Many homes were built from large bones and tusks driven into the ground and filled in with brush and turf. Try to imagine the strength it took to dig large pits, especially from the crudest of tools, to serve as traps for large prey. The clubs they carried were also heavy; knowing how to wield one could be the difference between life and death.

If a hunter had to roam far from home, he might also be required to carry a large section of the carcass many miles in order to feed the rest of the tribe. Antelope, bison, and reindeer weighing up to 200 pounds would have to be butchered, dragged, or otherwise transported to the main campsite. Nautilus machines hadn't yet arrived on the scene, there were no chiropractors available, and BenGay® had not been discovered yet, making strength development a necessary prerequisite for survival and injury prevention.

Finally, primitive man often lifted and transported huge rocks to be used for tools, weapons, and creating barriers. Anthropologists surmise that artificial dams with funnel-like rock intakes were built in large streams in order to trap fish, which could then be easily speared. Stone sculptures also required great strength and here also our ancestors were equal to the task, as archeological evidence indicates.

For the modern counterpart, strength can promote increased stress tolerance in the following ways:

1. A greater proportion of muscle to fat will decrease the effort (energy) required during normal everyday tasks. Fatigue is less likely to occur.
2. Posture is improved, promoting a better self-image. Studies on weightlifting frequently show substantial gains in self-confidence.
3. Strength development decreases the risk of injury since injuries usually result from sudden demands placed on weak muscles, tendons, and ligaments.
4. Throwing some weights around is better than throwing *your* weight around. Many has been the time I took out my anger pumping iron, after which I was relaxed enough to put a problem in its proper perspective and deal with it rationally.

Professionals like police, firefighters, and others required to exhibit sudden all-out bursts of energy should incorporate strength training. Statistics are substantiating fewer work-related injuries due to strength development, especially injuries to the lower spine.

I recommend you spend 25 percent of your total workout time on strength-building exercises at least three times per week.

Some experts advocate free weights, some advocate suspended weights. Generally speaking, free weights are better for development of posture since they work many antigravity muscle groups simultaneously. For the average individual this may have more transfer effect since it tends to resemble the stresses required of lifting objects in our day-to-day world. It is often difficult to get good leverage when lifting or manipulating objects in our environment. However, if you are training for a specific sport, event, or activity where skill may be enhanced by specifically isolating certain muscle groups, then suspended weights may offer a distinct advantage. Further, the chances of injury are apt to be less when using suspended weights than with free weights, which give the lifter a better mechanical advantage.

I use a combination of both. Remember how I trained specific muscle groups that were involved in climbing the building using Nautilus® machines. I use free weights when working many areas like my abdominal oblique or the pectoral muscles of my chest. My advice to you is to experiment, but don't neglect your cardiovascular fitness. As Dr. Jack Wilmore, noted exercise physiologist, says, "We don't die from lack of strength, we die from poor circulation." Almost half of all firefighters in three major cities died not from work-related hazards but from heart attacks and heart disease. Both forms of exercise, as well as flexibility (static stretching) exercises can stressproof you enormously and make life more enjoyable. A good-looking physique is a definite social attribute and can open many doors.

Testing Your Exercise Tolerance

Now it's time to test yourself, to see just how fit you are. Find a stable bench or platform 12 inches high. This platform can be constructed using a 12 inch cardboard box filled with books. Many kitchen stepstools are about this height.

Test of Heart/Lung Fitness

Directions: Stand before the bench. Begin by stepping upon the bench with one foot and bringing the other foot up. Then reverse this sequence as you step down. Step to the count of four to create a nice smooth rhythm. The proper cadence is 30 steps per minute. Your body should be erect when you step onto the bench. There is no rule regarding which foot you should lead with, nor is there any requirement to alternate the feet period-ically. This is left up to your own choice. I recommend alternating lead foot periodically. Continue to step at this prescribed cadence for three minutes or until you feel you must stop because of exhaustion. As soon as you stop, sit down and remain seated and quiet throughout the pulse counts. Take your pulse between 1 and 1½ minutes after the exercise test is completed and write down the number of heart beats. SCORING:

$$\text{Stress Tolerance Score} = \frac{\text{Duration of Exercise in secs.} \times 100}{5.5 \times \text{Pulse Count for 1 to 1½ Minutes after Exercise}}$$

Compare your score using the following norms: 0-50, poor; 50-65, fair; 65-80, average; 80-90, good; 90 and over, excellent.

Those who scored below average on stress tolerance should be able to improve their endurance by adhering to the rules given in chapter 13.

Be sure to develop a well-rounded, sound, progressive program of aerobic exercise, strength training, and slow stretching exercises for flex-ibility. Then, after a month or two, begin to observe how easily you handle the events in your life which seemed to weigh you down. You won't need your spear anymore.

> When I was smoking four packs of cigarettes a day, drinking ⅕th of Scotch every day, and weighed 300 pounds and hadn't exercised in 15 years, nobody said I was crazy. Now I'm one of the healthiest humans on this planet (Ran from New York to Los Angeles), and people question my health and mental attitude. If I ever came close to being crazy it was during those times when I was abusing myself in nightclubs.—DICK GREGORY (Civil rights activist and author)

CHAPTER 5
Selected References

California Nexus Foundation. "Corporate Health Promotion Programs." *A Progress Report*. San Francisco, Calif, May 1, 1983.

Chen, Moon S., Jr. "Wellness in the Workplace." *Review of the Literature, Health Values, Achieving High Level Wellness*. Vol. 6, No. 5, Sept–Oct, 1982.

DeVries, Herbert A. "Tranquilizer Effect of Exercise: A Critical Re-view." *Physician and Sportsmedicine*, Vol. 9, No. 11, November 1981, pp. 47–53.

Eyer, Joseph. *Hypertension as a Disease of Modern Society*, Chapter 7 from Stress and Survival, (ed.) Charles Garfield. C.V. Mosby, 1979.

Paffenbarger, Ralph S. *Physical Activity and Fatal Heart Attack: Protection or Selection?*, Chapter 3 from Exercise in Cardiovascular Health and Disease, (ed.) Ezra Amsterdam. Yorke Medical Books, 1977.

Nutrition: Discover the Primitive Diet

A Backward Glance

Our earliest ancestors lived primarily on berries, nuts, seeds, and roots, though insects like grasshoppers and ants provided an occasional welcome delicacy. As the use of tools developed they became more daring, were much less foragers of the land and could roam farther in search of food.

To bring down quarry early hunters used clubs, spears, darts, deadfalls (driving animals over cliffs) camouflaged pits, snares, nets, and weirs. Evidence from the Ambrona Valley in Spain provides interesting insights into how they obtained food. Using grass fires, bands of two or more tribes would unite (a rare occasion) to drive a herd of elephants into a mud bog. There the sheer weight of the animal would sink it to its knees at which point it was quite helpless. Then they would dispatch the animal with large rocks and spears then butcher it. Invention of the bow made things a lot easier, since they could kill their prey from long range.

Then came the domestication of plants and primitive people became less nomadic. The basic pattern of meat from the kill and vegetables from the soil continued for thousands of years with innumerable variations based on the land, the climate, and other geographical considerations. Primitive man's high fiber diet and grainy foods like seeds kept his teeth clean and healthy. Jaw bones recovered from archeological digs support this statement as well as dental analysis of primitive tribes currently residing in undeveloped areas of the world.

The Current Situation

The human animal of today no longer worries about the risks of a wild beast attack. He worries about the risks of a " Big-Mac attack." The fast-food industry of today stands in sharp contrast to the dietary patterns of our ancestors, and for that matter, even our grandparents of seventy years ago.

Our modern diet is extremely low in fiber, but high in salt, sugar, and fat. One prominent nutrition authority proposes that we follow a dietary program in which 10 percent of our calories come from fat, 10 percent from protein, and 80 percent from complex carbohydrates (whole grains, fruits, and vegetables). I believe this is an excellent idea. This is probably not too different from how primitive man ate, as best we can determine. The only problem here is one of practicality. Most people are not skilled enough to analyze how much fat, protein, and carbohydrate is in every bite of food they eat. Only nutritionists can do this, unless one carries a nutrition textbook around, which is one reason why many people have difficulty following that diet.

But, there is another reason. We live in the age of speed. Hurry, hurry, hurry. Instant this and instant that, and the modern food industry caters to this convenience need very well. Also, many of us are living very boring, unstimulating lives. And so the modern food industry meets us halfway here also, providing foods not so much geared toward nutritional needs as appealing to our taste, sight, and smell. They know the "snap, crackle, and pop," the sound of the fizz, and the package design will have strong psychological impact.

You, the consumer, can change this. The food industry is only catering to your misguided senses. Go back and see how you scored on the nutrition portion of the Life Risk Questionnaire in Chapter 1. What was your score? Let's see if you can improve your risk behaviors after reading this chapter.

The average American in 1900 ate ten pounds of sugar a year. Today, that figure is 110 pounds per year. This amounts to two and a half pounds per week per person. Most of it is hidden. For example, Heinz catsup is 28.9 percent sugar, nondairy coffee creamer is 65.4 percent sugar, cherry-flavored Jello is 82.6 percent sugar, and many ready-to-eat breakfast cereals contain 60 to 70 percent sugar. The average American consumed 410 twelve-ounce cans of soft drinks in 1981. The average American consumes 40 to 50 percent of the diet as fat calories. One survey indicated that the typical American meal taken from a restaurant menu contained a whopping 70 percent of the total calories in the form of fat. A study conducted at the University of California to determine the adult intake of eight nutrients revealed that the percentage of people consuming less than two-thirds of the RDA (Recommended Daily Allowance) showed that for all nutrients, deficiencies ranged from 5 percent for protein to 60 percent for calcium. Another study on children revealed similar results. On top of this, approximately 62 percent of Americans are considered overweight. No wonder everyone complains of too much stress!

My Quest for a High-Performance Diet

Prior to my high-risk activities, I thought I ate a fairly good diet. I didn't eat a lot of fatty foods, I avoided concentrated sugars, I avoided stimulants such as caffeine, and my alcohol intake was minimal. But survival required peak performance, so I began to gather as much information as I could regarding optimal performance and diet. The peak performance diet, it seems, is really the "primitive diet" (without the ants and the grasshoppers, of course).

I've listed below my nutritional suggestions for performing at high stress levels. It helped me a lot in dealing with the extreme fears and energy demands in the stunts and extreme sports I describe. I do not claim it will make you a superman, an allstar, or assure you victory in some sport. What it will do is give you more energy and thus an enhanced sense of well-being.

The Primitive Diet

Recommendation 1   Intake of dietary fiber should approximate 0.3 grams per each pound of body weight (40 to 60 grams/day)

Recommendation 2   80 percent of the daily protein intake should be of plant origin (whole grains, vegetables, nuts, seeds, etc.).

Recommendation 3   Eliminate stimulants (caffeine), alcohol, concentrated sugars, and unneeded drugs whenever possible.

Recommendation 4   Five or six feedings per day are preferred to the typical three large meals.

Recommendation 5   Supplement your diet with those specific nutrients required during specific high stress situations.

Now I will elaborate on each of these points, listing the recommendation, the scientific rationale, and basic applications.

Increase Fiber Intake to 40 to 60 Grams/Day

Scientific Rationale: If you did nothing else except try to follow this recommendation (and used common sense), you would find your health measurably improved for the following reasons, which have all been documented in studies on fiber intake.

1. Rapid food transit. Since fiber is the nondigestible portion of the plant, it assists in the passage of food through the intestine. This transit time, as it is called, takes less than one day when fiber intake is 40 or more grams/day. On the typical American refined food diet of less than 10 grams, transit time may be up to three days. This extra time allows more toxic wastes to build up in the intestinal tract, causing flatulence (gas), and a variety of other problems. One study found that patients treated with bran fiber (46 grams) for a week prior to abdominal surgery were able to resume normal bowel functions in half the time as those fed a normal hospital diet.

How do you know what your transit time is? Eat two or three tablespoons of kernel corn without chewing. Record the time this is done. The corn serves as a marker, so don't vary your normal eating pattern during this self-experiment. Watch from then on for evidence of the kernels in the stools. The total time they remain in your body is the "transit time:" 12 to 18 hours is ideal; 24 hours is good; and as this time extends to 40 or 50 hours, the likelihood of digestive problems (including cancer) increases.

2. High-fiber diets reduce the incidence of hemorrhoids, diverticulitis, diverticulosis, colon cancer, and other digestive problems. A ten-year study of 871 middle-aged men (*Lancet,* Sept. 4, 1982) revealed that those eating less than 37 grams per day had four times the rate of heart disease and three times the rate of cancer as those who ate more than 37 grams per day.

Dr. Paul Dudley White, after visiting the Hunza people in the Himalayas in 1964 and testing a group of men between 90 and 110 years old, found not a single person with any sign of coronary disease, high blood pressure, or high cholesterol. They eat at least 100 grams of fiber per day. Most of this comes from coconuts, chapattis (coursely ground grain made into a patty), apricots, raw fruits, vegetables, and nuts. They do not worship money, they worship apricot trees. Sally DeVore, in *The Appetites Of Man,* writes,

> They are very happy people. There is no crime, no police, no jails, no army, no hunger, and no distress. . . . Divorce exists but is extremely rare. If a wife cannot budget her food to stretch through the winter, the husband may get a divorce . . . the embarrassment is too much for him to handle.

3. High-fiber diets reduce the incidence of varicose veins, which can result from straining due to constipation.

4. Diets high in fiber improve glucose metabolism and have been shown to maintain the blood sugar level within more normal ranges. Hypoglycemia (low blood sugar), and diabetes are less likely. Insulin requirements in diabetics have been reduced or eliminated on high fiber diets. Such diets are now an essential component in the management of diabetic patients. Dr. Jack Davidson, Director of the Diabetes Unit at Emory University Medical School, has found that, after 11,000 patients evaluated over a twelve-year period, 80 percent improved much better on a high-fiber diet of fruits, vegetables, and skim milk than those treated with drugs.

In another study, 95 grams of fiber per day improved diabetic control of both noninsulin- and insulin-dependent patients whereas 20 grams did not. (*British Medical Jour.* May 29, 1982).

5. Fiber absorbs bile acids, reducing fat absorption. Dr. James Anderson, Professor of Medicine at the University of Kentucky College of Medicine, found that blood cholesterol was lowered by as much as 30 percent by eating very high-fiber diets. The best high-fiber foods for lowering colesterol are oat products, all varieties of beans, and unpeeled fruits. Scientists believe that the water soluble fibers found in such foods form a

gel around the cholesterol molecule during digestion and entrap it so it can't be absorbed into the bloodstream to form fat deposits.

Studies at the University of Kentucky have shown that ½ cup a day of oat bran mixed into the typical American diet can lower the serum cholesterol by 25 percent in as little as 10 days. Wow! That's better than the drugs used to lower cholesterol, without the side effects.

Medical studies on the !Kung San of the Kalahari Desert in Botswana show serum cholesterols of 120 mg.% (and no significant variation by age). Such values are rare indeed in western society and are attributed to the large amounts of fiber in their diets.

6. High-fiber diets have been shown to aid weight control very effectively. The extra bulk created satisfies the appetite at lower caloric levels. You lose weight without necessarily having to count calories, although such restriction is still advised. Researchers at the University of Alabama, after teaching obese people to select high-fiber foods without worrying about calories, found that those on such diets ate almost 1,500 fewer calories per day than another group of obese people. The high-fiber group always felt full and satisfied. Counting calories is a poor gauge to nutritional status. We should focus on counting intake of daily fiber in grams.

7. In order to satisfy the requirements of a 40 to 60 gram fiber intake per day, you'll eat more whole foods since fiber is only found in appreciable amounts in fruits, vegetables, and natural grains. This almost insures an adequate intake of vitamins A, B and C complex, E, minerals like potassium, calcium, and iron, and other nutrients often removed in modern food processing.

8. High-fiber diets promote healthy teeth and gums because of the cleansing action and chewing required of fibrous, grainy foods. The incidence of tooth misalignment in young children has drastically increased in recent years and has been blamed on soft diets that require minimal chewing. One study found that by age 14, over one-third of the average child's teeth were decayed and by 17 years of age, 68 percent had advanced stages of periodontal disease.

Our primitive ancestors did lots of crunching and griding food on their molars to break down the roots, nuts, grains, and seeds they ate. They did rather well without dentists. Herman Melville, commenting on the Marquesan Islanders in the South Pacific in 1841, said:

> Nothing in the appearance of the islanders struck me more forcibly than the whiteness of their teeth, they were more beautiful than ivory itself. The jaws of the oldest among them were much better than those of the youth of civilized countries. This marvelous whiteness of teeth is to be ascribed to the pure vegetable diet of these people and the uninterrupted healthiness of their natural mode of life.

Somehow, this happened even without Ultra-Brite or Close Up toothpaste.

Incidently, after we "civilized" them, we nearly destroyed these people, their population dropping from 120,000 to 1,000 by 1920, the result of our modern degenerative diseases.

9. A high-fiber diet, (50 grams), greatly increases your intake of silicon, an often overlooked and valuable nutrient for protecting against arthritis and atherosclerosis, as autopsy studies on humans suggests. Silicon improves the strength of bones, tendons, hair, nails, and the cell membrane itself.

10. Finally, a high-fiber diet may offer protection against appendicitis. One of the world's foremost authorities on fiber, Dr. Dennis Burkitt, a member of the British Medical Research Council, long ago described a pattern related to this problem.

> In less developed communities virtually everywhere, appendicitis was a rarity; more and more, as those communities developed and shifted to Western refined diets, or as natives moved from the less developed to the more developed, appendicitis increased and became common. . . . At the Korle Bu Hospital in Accra, Ghana, there were less than 10 operations a year for appendicitis in the 1940's; by 1960 there were 70; by 1965, 145. In Nairobi, Kenya, in 1937, in a series of 1,000 autopsies on Africans, only a single case of appendicitis was found; by the late 1960's more than 150 cases a year were being admitted for surgery.

Application of a High-Fiber Diet

Because fiber is so important, I've provided a list of high-fiber foods. Remember, the individual amount of fiber taken in grams per day should be 0.3 times your weight in pounds. For example, a 150 lb. man would need 0.3 times 150 or 45 grams fiber/day. On this diet your energy level will increase and you'll learn how stimulating it can be to crunch and chew once again.

Dietary Fiber in Foods We Eat

Food	Portion Size	Grams/Fiber
High fiber and bran cereals	½ cup	up to 13.5
Baked beans	½ cup	8.3
Apple	1 large	7.4
Broccoli (cooked)	1 med. stalk	7.4
Shredded coconut	1 pc. 2"x2"x½"	6.1
Dried fruit	½ cup	3.0–6.0
Brown Rice (raw)	½ cup	5.8
Spinach, cooked	½ cup	5.7
Figs, dried	5	5.6
Guava and mangos	1 med.	5.6

Food	Portion Size	Grams/Fiber
Garbanzos	½ cup	5.5
Blackberries	½ cup	5.3
Almonds	¼ cup	5.1
Kidney beans	½ cup	4.5
Azuki beans	½ cup	4.3
Cabbage, shredded	½ cup	4.3
Peas (cooked)	½ cup	4.2
White beans	½ cup	4.2
Pinto beans	½ cup	4.0
Banana	1 med.	4.0
Corn	½ cup	3.9
Potato	1 med.	3.9
Pear	1 med.	3.8
Millet	½ cup	3.7
Lentils	½ cup	3.7
Lima beans (cooked)	½ cup	3.5
Sweet potato	1 med.	3.5
Sunflower seeds	½ cup	3.0
Chopped peanuts	¼ cup	2.9
Cornflakes	1 cup	2.8
Orange	1 med.	2.6
Raisins	¼ cup	2.5
Artichoke	1 med.	2.5
Brussels sprouts	4	2.4
Dates	10 med.	2.3
Whole wheat bread	1 slice	2.3
Apricots	3 med.	2.3
Raw carrots	1 med.	2.3
Beets	½ cup	2.1
Peaches	1 med.	2.1
Zucchini (raw)	½ cup	2.0
String beans (raw)	½ cup	1.9
Puffed wheat	1 cup	1.8
Tomato (raw)	1 med.	1.8
Barley (raw)	½ cup	1.6
Miller's bran	1 tablespoon	1.6
Onions (cooked)	½ cup	1.6
Strawberries	½ cup	1.6

Food	Portion Size	Grams/Fiber
Coconut (shredded)	½ cup	1.6
Walnuts (chopped)	¼ cup	1.6
Sesame seeds	½ cup	1.5
Wheat germ	½ cup	1.3
Asparagus (chopped)	½ cup	1.2
Cherries	10	1.1
Cauliflower (raw)	½ cup	1.0
Pineapple	1¾" slice	1.0
Asparagus	4 med. spears	0.9
White bread	1 slice	0.8
Celery (raw)	1 stalk	0.7
Onions (raw, chopped)	½ cup	0.6

The question may arise, why did I choose 40 to 60 grams of fiber per day as the minimal amount? To some degree this was an arbitrary figure, although if one takes a good look at the scientific literature, I seriously doubt that you will find any evidence that cancer of the digestive system, heart disease, arthritis, adult-onset diabetes, osteoporosis, or any of our modern diseases occur where fiber intake of this amount has been followed continuously. Dr. Peter Van Soest, a nutritionist at Cornell University, after twenty-five years of research on fiber intake, says: "We've done a lot of research on intakes of 40, 50, and 60 grams of fiber a day and its been very successful."

Adding a small amount of bran fiber is okay as long as you are not simply adding fiber to a refined, overprocessed diet. The recommended amount should come from whole foods. Remember, the concept of keeping track of your fiber intake is to get you in the habit of automatically eating the right kind of foods, more complex carbohydrates, and putting the crunch back into eating. Don't do something crazy like live on bananas or peanuts.

The illustration on page 74, "The Handy Five," will serve as a reminder to help you obtain a variety of foods with an adequate intake of fiber. The illustration shows clearly what foods are in which groups. On a daily basis, you should have at least three helpings from each of the first four groups— fruits; vegetables; grains, including pasta; and nuts and legumes (beans and peas). From the fifth group—animal—at least two helpings daily will help promote optimal health. This group includes meat, fish, eggs, and dairy products such as butter and cheese. Fruits should be eaten with the peel if possible, vegetables raw or slightly steamed, and grains with the husk intact to add fiber content.

Those who expend more energy (calories) per day will need even more fiber, perhaps even as much as 80 grams a day. Dr. Van Soest offers these suggestions for a high fiber diet:

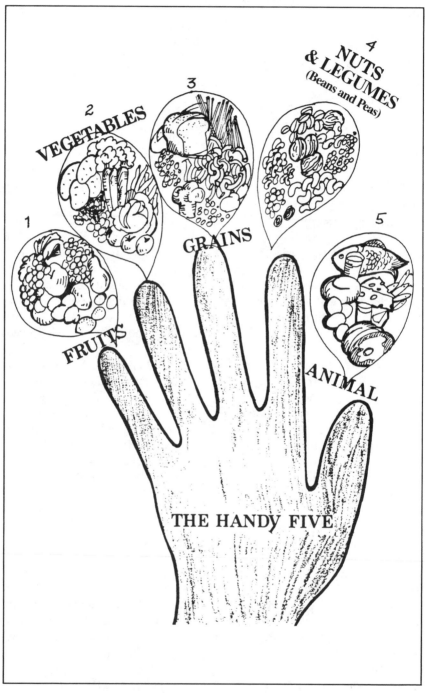

1. Don't add excessive amounts of fiber to the diet abruptly. Allow at least three weeks to build up to this level. (This is extremely important. Otherwise you likely will experience various digestive problems, the result of not giving your body the time necessary to adapt to the new regimen. Those people with a history of digestive disorders, like ulcerative colitis, should consult with their physician before starting this diet.)
2. Be flaky. Coarse particle size is most important. If you take wheat bran and mill it to flour fineness, it loses its capacity to speed passage of food through the intestinal tract. Stone-ground flours, whether wheat, oats, barley, or rye are better because they are large and flaky in size.
3. When reading labels, look for the words "dietary fiber," not "crude fiber." There can be a big difference between the two. Dietary fiber gives an accurate description of fiber content.

Take Protein Requirements from Plant Sources

Scientific rational: Studies cntinue to demonstrate that
1. Diets high in animal protein are associated with heart and blood vessel diseases because of the high saturated fat content such diets contain. This finding is well documented.
2. While providing protein, the biological food value of meat is substantially less than that of many vegetable proteins, especially when vegetable proteins are properly combined. (You will learn how shortly.)
Application of More Vegetable Proteins How much protein do you need? You need approximately 1 gram of protein for every 2.5 pounds of body weight. Protein is used for repair and maintenance of tissue, formation of hormones, and antibodies (which protect us against disease).

A 100-pound woman would need 40 grams of protein per day and a 200-pound man would need 80 grams of protein per day. If 80 percent of this is from nonmeat sources, then the woman needs to get 32 grams of protein from vegetable, nut, and grain sources, and the man, 64 grams per day of nonmeat protein to meet this recommendation.

Do I expect you to go around counting grams of protein? Not necessarily. Once again, recall the previous recommendation for 40–60 grams of fiber. If you'll adhere to this recommendation and use common sense, you should have little difficulty fulfilling this second recommendation. For example, note the protein in the following foods.

Protein Composition of some High Fiber Foods

Food	Portion Size	Grams of Protein
Garbanzos	½ cup	20.5

Food	Portion Size	Grams of Protein
Pumpkin seeds	½ cup	20.3
Sunflower seeds	½ cup	17.0
Pinto beans	½ cup	15.0
Wheat germ	½ cup	14.0
Almonds	½ cup	13.5
Black walnuts	½ cup	13.0
Millet	½ cup	12.0
Azuki beans	½ cup	11.0
Soybeans	½ cup	10.0
Barley	½ cup	10.0
Brown rice	½ cup	8.0
Black Eyed peas	½ cup	8.0
Cornmeal	½ cup	5.5
Raw wheat bran	½ cup	4.5
Figs	5 med.	4.3
Whole grain breads	1 slice	2.5
White (refined) bread	1 slice	0.9

All these foods except white bread are high in fiber. Now you are doing two things at once, getting your high fiber intake and meeting your protein requirement. You are also saving a lot on your food bill, as I will point out later.

The remaining protein can be met with milk (8 grams/8 oz. glass), eggs (6 grams each), and white meats like fish, turkey and chicken (with the skin removed). Avoid frying or *any* use of heated oils. This practice produces free radicals, which have been implicated in atherosclerosis and premature aging.

Are you bored with meats like beef and chicken? Well then, try some buffalo meat. According to data from the U.S. Department of Agriculture, it's lower in cholesterol and higher in both protein and thiamine than beef and many varieties of fish. For more information call the American Buffalo Association at 307/587-4895.

By the way, how about that much misaligned egg? Not one scientific study has ever shown that eating eggs causes heart disease. In fact, one group of researchers found blood cholesterol increased significantly only in smokers who ate three eggs per day. So what about Humpty Dumpty? I have my own version.

> Humpty Dumpty sat on a wall,
> He was a good ol' egg who befriended cholesterol.
> But the American Heart Association,
> In spite of his fame,
> For heart disease, had decided he was to blame.

They gathered a committee who shoved Humpty off the wall,
Poor innocent Humpty took a great fall.
But all the King's horses and all the King's men
Knew the evidence was scant he'd committed a sin.
With the help of some chemists who explained Lecithin,
They finally put Humpty Dumpty back together again.
And the American Dairy Association lived happily ever after!

Lecithin is a phospholipid which acts naturally as an emulsifier; that is, it breaks fat up into tiny particles to assist absorption of the fats by the cells. Animal studies have shown that lecithin can dissolve atheromatous placques (fat deposits) in blood vessels. Additional research needs to be done.

Smaller, More Frequent Meals

Scientific rationale: Studies have shown that such eating behaviors result in

1. Better regulation of blood sugar levels, which takes excess stress off the pancreas (to produce insulin). This reduces the incidence and severity of hypoglycemia and diabetes. Because the blood sugar does not fluctuate widely on smaller, more frequent meals, mood swings tend to be minimized, resulting in a more stable personality. Studies on young school children have revealed that disruptive behaviors are better controlled in this fashion, that is, by taking eating breaks between meal time. Studies on ancient cultures reveal that these people follow such eating patterns, eating often throughout the day rather than gorging themselves two or three times a day. The modern eating pattern is no doubt a byproduct of our structured work day.

2. Studies show there is less fat absorption when the same daily calories are eaten in six feedings rather than three. This reduces the likelihood of fat particles forming placques on the interior walls of blood vessels.

3. The problem of overeating is reduced since appetite is better controlled. Studies show people tend to consume fewer calories per day when they are allowed to eat more often. This ad-lib eating pattern is called "graying."

Application—How to Beat the System   Take foods to work with you that you can munch on between meals or during break: raisins, dates, figs, sunflower seeds, apples, bananas, other fruits, and whole grain crackers. Eat apples with the peel, oranges, grapefruits, and potatoes with the peel. Sunflower and pumpkin seeds come in convenient little pouches you can keep in your desk. Put dates in plastic bags.

If you do not have a desk job so you can keep food out of sight, take carrot sticks to munch on at breaks, or at the very least, buy something nutritious like yogurt (if you want a sweet taste, get regular yogurt and add orange juice concentrate, carob drops, a small amount of fructose, or raisins).

If you don't have a desk job, don't get breaks, someone is always watching you, and you are not a female so you can sneak into your purse under the pretense of putting on makeup, do this: Tell your boss you found out you have bad kidneys and you need to use the restroom often. If you carry a hard-boiled egg or granola bar in your pocket it will not be conspicuous. You can wolf it down when you reach your destination. If you get caught, go ahead and blame it on me, I'll take the rap. But be sure and tell him I said you'll be able to concentrate and work better because of this strategy. If the boss fires you, be a positive risk taker. You will be healthier somewhere else anyway.

Eliminate Harmful Stimulants and Drugs

The list includes coffee, non-herbal teas, alcohol, and all foods with purified (concentrated) sugars.

Scientific rational: Four or more cups of coffee per day are associated with a 3 to 4 times greater-than-normal occurrence of pancreatic cancer, and twice the normal rate of stomach cancer. Coffee also increases the incidence of abnormal heart rhythms, a condition one certainly wants to avoid when peak performance is desired.

Studies have also shown that it interferes with what is called *complex reaction time*; that is, the time taken to react to a stimulus when faced with several choices. This implies that decision making under high-stress conditions may be impaired when high doses of caffeine are consumed.

I've had dietitians tell me there's no proof that coffee in small amounts is going to harm someone. I disagree. Studies now show that some people are caffeine sensitive and even a small amount can send the blood pressure rocketing in such people. As a student of neurophysiology, I learned that caffeine acts similarly to an amphetamine. It excites the central nervous system. This results in accelerated heart rate, elevated blood pressure, release of potentially damaging hormones in the blood, and liberation of fats into the blood (called free fatty acids). None of these actions are desirable. Like any amphetamine, it hastens the depletion of our energy reserves. This may result in lowered stress tolerance, especially over a period of years. This may be one reason why Dr. Hans Selye, the "father of stress", maintained that caffeine causes premature aging.

Recent research conducted at John Hopkins University and the National Institute of Arthritis, Metabolism, and Digestive Diseases discovered that caffeine interferes with the action of adenosine, a naturally occurring chemical we all possess. Adenosine acts as a natural tranquilizer, which is released when we are highly stressed. Caffeine, by blocking the release of this chemical in the brain, prevents the natural relaxation effect from taking place. So, if you want to be a "coffee achiever," give that some thought.

One study found that coffee taken within one hour of a meal inhibited iron absorption, a nutrient that plays a key role in the transportation of oxygen (*American Journal of Clinical Nutrition,* Vol. 37, 1983). Dr. Roy Matthew, at Vanderbilt University, found that blood flow to the brain was reduced by 25 percent from drinking the caffeine contained in two cups of freshly brewed coffee.

As for white refined sugar, much can be said, and the literature is replete with studies on its hazards if you look in the right places. An excellent book on the subject is Dr. John Yudkin's *Sweet and Dangerous.* Dr. Yudkin, a physician and biochemist, has investigated this topic for many years.

Sugar increases both calcium and magnesium excretion and excess intake can create depletion of the trace mineral chromium, a nutrient extremely necessary for controlling blood-sugar level. Increased sugar consumption also increases the need for thiamine (B_1). A deficiency in this vitamin can result in neurotic behavior, hysteria, sleep disturbances, and other asocial behaviors usually treated with drugs or counseling. Needless to say, refined sugar decreases your stress tolerance enormously if you take it long enough. One study indicated that sugar decreased by 50 percent the ability of white cells to destroy bacteria. Since it is our white cells that provide resistance to diseases, anything that suppresses their function should be avoided at all costs.

The Eskimos living in their natural habitats are one of the most stress-resistant people in the entire world. They consume huge amounts of dietary fat in the form of seal oil. Yet, left to themselves, they develop heart disease at one-tenth the rate of Urbanized Americans. When we westernize them however, things change. As Sally DeVore writes,

> When they increase their intake of sugars and starches in the form of refined and manufactured foods, decay increases as much as 150%. Urban eskimos now have about the worst teeth in the world. In addition, cancer, arthritis, and other degenerative diseases are seen where none existed before. The Eskimo loses his natural immunity that heretofore protected him.

What was it about the diet that protected them so well? The Eskimo diet contains two-and-a-half-times the fiber of our diets, five times the calcium, and more than ten times the amounts of vitamins A and D found in the American diet. Also, there is a substance found in seal oil called EPA (eicosapentanoic acid). It's believed this substance is incorporated into the fat of arteries and membranes, causing the release of prostaglandins, substances that stimulate repair of the arterial wall. In one study, EPA was shown to lower cholesterol from 188 to 162 mg.%.

What about alcohol: Why am I against it? In very small amounts it probably isn't harmful, especially naturally fermented beverages like beer and wine, which do contain some nutrients. The problem is, it is a mood-altering substance; as such, it can become addictive. Even if it is not used in excessive amounts, it winds up replacing more desired calories like those from fruit juices. I can see you snarling right now. "He's taking my sources of pleasure away". No, not really. A glass of Perrier with ½ lemon or lime will provide the fizz to tickle your tongue. Once you've quit drinking all alcohol for several months and drink ample water and fruit juices, you won't even want it anymore.

As for drugs, don't get the idea I'm talking about illegal drugs and so you're exempt. The large majority of drug abusers in this country are doing it legally, taking pain killers, cold pills, tranquilizers and similar drugs. They "doctor-shop," rotating physicians so they can continue to get the refills to support their addictions. Such drugs can wreak nutritional havoc with the body, upsetting the normal mineral balances needed for high energy levels and peak performance.

Application: Find Substitute Stimulants   Begin to read labels. Avoid foods that contain sugar. Even as I write today, I've just received a "free" bag of cookies in the mail and "a chance to win $10,000 cash in the Taste-of-Home Sweepstakes". The squirrels will love the cookies but I'll send in the Sweepstakes. What would they do with $10,000 anyway?

Herbal teas can be quite stimulating to those in need of caffeine substitutes without the negative side effects. Teas like Ginseng (Siberian, Korean), Peppermint, Mate (South American), Sarsparilla (Domestic), Ginger, Cinnamon Rose, Orange Spice, and many others can satisfy the craving for a stimulant.

Crob is a powder that looks, tastes, and almost smells like chocolate. It is made from a tree and is a protein, which can substitute well as a hot morning beverage to replace coffee.

Whenever your sweet tooth craves something, eat fruits. They are high in fructose which releases insulin in a much slower, controlled fashion than sucrose (table sugar).

Dr. William Evans at Tufts University compared blood sugar responses of three groups before, during, and after a 30-minute treadmill run. One group used water, one group used glucose, and another used fructose. He found depletion of muscle glycogen (muscle fuel) and wide blood-sugar fluctuations in the glucose group. The athletes who consumed fructose maintained more stable blood-sugar levels and had significantly more muscle glycogen left after the 30-minute run than did the glucose group. Athletes who had water only fared better than the glucose group.

In recipes calling for sugar, use concentrated orange juice. You'll get a good dose of vitamin C to boot.

If you don't have access to an icebox at work, freeze a banana the night before and take it to work in some foil. By around 10:00 it should be nice and soft and ready to eat. Another delight is a Carob Crunch, a rice cake coated with carob. Most health food stores carry these.

Use Supplementation when Needed

Scientific rational: Many studies show that some nutrients are needed in greater amounts to combat elevated stress levels. These include especially vitamins C, B Complex, pantothenic acid, and many others, according to the specific stressor. Examples follow.

Use of the birth control pill has been shown to have a marked effect on the body's need for and use of trace minerals copper, zinc, and iron, as well as vitamins B_2, B_6, B_{12}, and folic acid. Approximately 95 percent of serum copper is bound to a copper binding protein ceruloplasmin, which is synthesized in the liver at an accelerated rate because of the pill.

Studies on vitamin C show that, in megadoses, it prevents the spread of cancer. Dr. Linus Pauling says it does this by inhibiting the enzyme hyaluronidase, a substance that breaks down the collagen (cellular cement) in normal cell membranes, making it vulnerable to infiltration by cancer cells. As the authors of *Life Extension*, in their summary on vitamin C and cancer, state:

> Vitamin C is itself poisonous to certain cancer cells at levels tolerated by normal cells; probably its major actions are to activate the T-cell immune system and to increase your body's production of interferon, an anti-virus and anti-cancer chemical.

They cite the work of Pauling and Cameron, who found that life expectancies of cancer patients given 10 grams orally increased more than four times that of controls not given C.

Studies on athletes have shown that those taking vitamin C have fewer injuries and one study concluded: "Using one gram of vitamin C daily, the subjects could perform significantly more work during the ascorbic acid period" (*Anabolism*, Sept., 1982).

Several studies have shown that the stress of surgery can result in drops of from 18 to 42 percent in serum vitamin C.

Another study found that subjects who smoked (27 percent of our population smokes) 20 or more cigarettes per day required 140 mg. of vitamin C to compensate for the vitamin C destroyed by smoke. I take one gram of C per day and rarely suffer from colds.

The role of vitamin E in stress, is another example. Vitamin-E-supplemented animals could swim from two to five times as long before drowning as non-E-supplemented animals. Then there were the original experiments with race horses conducted at the Windfield Farms in Ontario, Canada. Given up to 5000 international units (I.U.) of E, the horses' winnings tripled within a year or two. The extensive research of Dr. Tom Cureton, then of the University of Illinois, showed that vitamin E enhanced endurance in middle-aged subjects. This claim was contested sharply by the FDA. Legal attempts to block the claim went all the way to the Illinois State Supreme Court, which ruled in favor of Dr. Cureton's extensive findings. Octocasanol is the endurance factor in vitamin E and can be obtained as a supplement in many health food stores.

Vitamin-E-supplemented diets accompanied the Apollo II crew on their historic moon voyage. Why? It was found that vitamin E's antioxidant properties prevented hemolytic anemia (destruction of the oxygen-carrying red blood cells), a side effect of breathing pure oxygen. Vitamin E is a free radical scavenger, which means it prevents premature aging. By protecting cell membranes, it potentiates the immune system (like vitamin C, selenium, and lecithin). I suggest 600 I.U./day, an amount shown to be safe and effective.

If vitamin supplements are so necessary, how is it people living in the uncivilized ("primitive") areas of the world seem to do quite well without them? The reason is simple; they don't have to deal with air, water, and food pollution, the hazards of the Pill, our fast pace of life, cigarettes, excessive alcohol consumption, and nutrient-deficient soils. There's another factor that is even more crucial. Since primitive people raised (or foraged) their own food, they did not suffer the loss of nutrients from storge, canning or freezing, time of transportation, washing (to remove pesticides), and cooking. For example, a raw potato will lose about half its vitamin C six weeks after harvest. It will lose another 25 percent after being peeled, cooked, and mashed. If it is reconstituted into potato flakes for quick preparation, it may wind up with only 8.6% of its original raw, fresh vitamin C content. Primitive peoples would have enjoyed the full vitamin C content (plus potassium, plus fiber from the peel) which their modern counterparts rarely do.

Dr. Emmanuel Cheraskin, in his book *Diet and Disease,* presents evidence that washing, along with preparation and cooking, can cause mineral losses of from 5 to 20 percent for phosphorus, calcium, and iron, as well as thiamine and niacin. Heat preparation can also destroy amino acids in the proteins, he points out.

Also, many food composition tables are outdated, that is, are not reliable indicators of the actual nutrient content.

Application: Nutritional Supplementation   There are three important things to remember in evaluating your need for nutritional supplementation.

First, a wide variety of conditions, some of which were mentioned, can create a need for additional nutrients. If you cannot at least make a concerted effort to follow the first two recommendations, supplementation seems even more necessary.

Second, any substance (vitamin or mineral) which increases the body's ability to use oxygen (vitamin E, etc.) should also enhance performance, since fatigue will be delayed. You should have more energy; you should be able to perform more work.

Third, since poor stress tolerance is related to almost every major disease, any substance that enhances the immune system is also going to increase your stress tolerance, since you will be less vulnerable to foreign organisms such as bacteria and viruses. Your immune system will be able to destroy them successfully.

Regarding the first point, it is my feeling everyone should take a high-potency vitamin-mineral tablet as a form of insurance. As the information presented indicates, our industrialized society and our pace of living seem to justify this conclusion.

Dr. Jeff Bland, Professor of Chemistry at the University of Puget Sound, and author of *Your Health Under Seige,* has found that vitamin C requirements may differ from person to person by a factor of 16, vitamin B_3 excretion by a factor of 4, and vitamin B_6 excretion by a factor of 35. Individual biochemical requirements are so variable, no single gauge can meet everyone's needs.

The RDA was established to serve as a guideline for "normal" people. It was established by the Food and Drug Administration based upon amounts slightly in excess of the typical American diet. The vitamin/mineral doses were not based upon extensive scientific analysis of our needs. If this had been the case, the amounts would be much higher. For example, Dr. Daphne Roe, at Cornell University, has found that women who exercise need at least twice the RDA levels for vitamin B_2. I have given many other examples already. Wellness doesn't imply maintenance doses, it implies optimal doses, and the FDA doesn't care about optimal.

As for point two, Vitamins C and E were mentioned as oxygen enhancers. Selenium and the phospholipid lecithin are believed to serve this function also. This is why lecithin is frequently used as a preservative, to prevent spoilage from oxidation of fats.

Dr. Linus Pauling recommends 2 to 3 grams per day of vitamin C. Dr. Bland recommends 1 gram per day, an amount which should be easily tolerated. Two notes of caution here. Build up slowly and once you are taking large doses, do not discontinue immediately. Gradually taper off to prevent a compromised immune system.

The vitamin B-complex group is involved in the release of energy from the cell. If you are under great stress, or consume a large amount of alcohol or refined sugar, then you may be deficient in the B-complex group.

As for the third point, good general nutrition (adequate protein, intake of needed vitamins and minerals) will maintain your immune system in good order. However, there is considerable research to suggest that certain vitamins in large amounts can offer additional protection. For example, vitamin A in large amounts seems to reduce vulnerability to cancer. However, this vitamin in large doses can be very toxic. There is a way to get around this problem. We can manufacture our own vitamin A if we have the precursor beta-carotene. Beta-carotene has been shown to reduce the incidence of lung cancer. If you follow recommendation #1 and eat plenty of fruits and vegetables, you will be getting a large intake of this nutrient.

Vitamin C, as already explained, seems to enhance the immune system. Besides promoting strength of the cell wall, it also increases the amount of interferon, a large protein in the blood that inactivates many viruses. Vitamin C in large amounts may also lower cholesterol, and decrease Chol/HDL ratios, thus lowering the risk of heart disease. (*Lancet,* Nov. 3, 1979).

For those who wish to be as scientific as possible in charting their intake of protein, fat, carbohydrate, fiber, vitamins and minerals in order to reach peak performance levels, I suggest utilizing the "Nutri-Check" system developed by Dr. Norge Jerome, a nutritional anthropologist, at K. U. Medical Center in K.C. It can also provide a lot of valuable information regarding eating behaviors (913-588-2791).

You will recall that I took 25 grams of vitamin C intravenously to help combat some of the stresses I faced. This was done under the supervision of a Dr. Charles Rudolph, a physician and Ph.D biochemist, who has a large practice in allergies and preventive medicine. We have also used this on several world-ranked endurance athletes with seemingly good results and no side effects. Still, this procedure should be considered experimental and *not* attempted without the supervision of a nutritionally competent physician.

Weight Control

Dr. Richard Lazarus in a year long research study, at the University of California at Berkeley, discovered that the little daily hassles are more closely linked to (and may have a greater effect on) our moods and our health than the major misfortunes of life. The number-one hassle, he found, was concern about weight. The number-two hassle was concern about health of a family member, and number 3 was concern about the rising prices of common goods. Now, think about this for a minute. Virtually every hassle can be helped by following the five recommendations. By avoiding refined, highly processed foods, and avoiding high-fat foods (red meats, hot dogs, lunch meats, fried foods, etc.) you will naturally begin to show a weight loss.

CAUTION: Weight loss without wellness enhancement is poor risk taking. In fact, the use of crash diets has been shown to result in a net gain of 105 percent the original weight. The rhythm method of girth control does not work.

Weight alone as an indicator of health is not reliable. The percentage of body fat is much more revealing. If you can sink slowly to the bottom of a swimming pool even with a full breath of air, your body fat percentage is 15 percent or lower. Those who pass this test have a higher stress

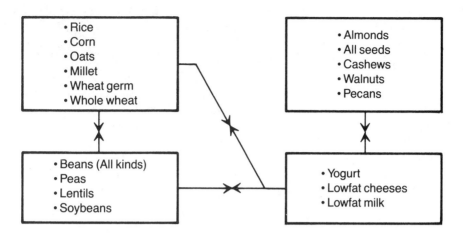

tolerance than those who can't. Why? Your heart has to work a lot harder, since fat requires its own circulation and yet is dead weight to be lugged around. You fatigue much more quickly. Besides the extra stress on the heart, the overfat person doesn't look as good, feels more social pressure, and tends to have a lower self-esteem. Therefore, under high-stress conditions they will often withdraw, only to experience hostility, anger, depression, or some other negative emotion. As for hassle number three, a high-fiber diet with 80 percent of the protein from vegetable sources will measurably reduce your monthly grocery bill. For example, a two-to-one combination of corn and beans will give you protein superior to meat at about 10 percent of the cost. The Chinese diet of brown rice, vegetables, and sprouts warmed lightly in a wok are inexpensive and easy to prepare. We have been conditioned to think we need to eat a large portion of meat at each meal. Use the above chart to make complete proteins.

To make a complete protein and add fiber to your diet, combine one food item from each box as the arrows show. Examples of these combinations include: Rice and bean casserole, bean burrito, baked beans and cornbread, macaroni and cheese, cereal with milk, or rice and cheese casserole.

Now I want to tell you about a roommate I had during my first year of graduate school. He lived on 50 cents per day. His dad sent him $6.00 per day food allowance, most of which went to make his payments on a color TV and his motorcycle. Yes, he survived quite well on 50 cents per day. What was his secret? He ate Purina Dog Chow—you know, the hard stuff. I remember his lugging a 50 pound bag of dog chow in, as I looked around the yard for the dog who was supposed to eat it! As a student of health his diet caused me great concern until I compared it with that of the dormitory students. The dog chow was loaded with protein, calcium, phosphorus, and other vitamins and minerals from the corn meal, wheat meal, soybeans, and other cereal grains. The dorm students ate a highly refined, starchy low-protein diet. Yes, Sam was getting more nutrition from the dog food. I did get him to take a vitamin C supplement, since dogs synthesize their C from carbohydrates, but humans cannot.

The most annoying part was being awakened at midnight listening to Sam crunching away on a midnight snack. It sounded like someone grinding nuts. We reached a good compromise, however. I agreed to put up with the late-night snacking as long as Sam agreed not to chase cars. Seriously . . . he had the whitest teeth on campus even if his jaws began to look like a bulldog from all the chewing. He claimed to have plenty of energy and he lost twenty pounds of fat.

Dr. Donald Davis, professor of chemistry at the University of California at Irvine, put rats on four different diets, composed of accepted staple foods. One group received an approximation of the urban American diet, consisting of white bread, sugar, eggs, milk, ground beef, cabbage, potatoes, tomatoes, oranges, apples, bananas, and coffee. The same diet was supplemented with thirteen trace elements for a second group. The third received Purina Rat Chow (which contains unrefined grains and fish meal fortified with vitamins and minerals), and the fourth got the rat chow diluted with sugar to provide 70 percent of the calories. It is no surprise to learn which diet resulted in optimal growth, size, and general health: the undiluted rat chow. The supplemented human diet was a close second with the others far behind.

I'm not implying we eat dog chow or rat chow. I mean we need to remind ourselves how primitive people ate, take a lesson from them, and to that add our superior knowledge regarding nutrition.

Risk Taking

Remember, every time you put something in your mouth you are throwing the dice. On the "Monopoly Board" of life, we all want to land on the good squares and have great things happen. But in this real-life game, our initial gift was not $1500 play money, but energy reserves that are determined to a large degree by what we eat. Remember, you have opponents in this game.

Perhaps wellness nutrition is best served by maintaining an attitude of suspicion. Your opponents can be rather misleading. For example, "2% low-fat milk" (by weight) sounds okay, right? You should know that 36 percent of the total calories are fat. Does that sound "low"? Beware the limericks, jingles, tongue twisters, and slogans, all blended together with special sauces and served on a sesame seed bun.

Eating nutritional foods (good moves) builds our reserves and eating junk food (poor moves) slowly depletes them. We aren't perfect. We will make mistakes. But if the good moves far exceed the bad ones, we are loading our dice; we will "Pass Go and Collect $200." We will win in this game of life.

Sample One-day Menu

The one-day menu on these pages illustrates the basic dietary recommendations I have listed. The requirement for protein was based on a 175-pound person. At 1 gram per 2.5 pounds, the protein needed is about 70 grams/day. About 80 percent of this amount comes from vegetable or plant sources, and the minimum 50 grams of fiber is also incorporated into the menu. Our one-day plan approximates 1800 to 2000 calories, yet provides the basic nutrients plus plenty of fiber.

Meal	Foods	Fiber (gr)	Protein (gr)
Breakfast	½ cup wheat bran cereal, ½ cup milk, 1 soft-boiled egg, 1 slice whole-grain bread, fruit juice	10	16
Snack	½ cup dried fruit, ¼ cup almonds or granola bar	6	7
Lunch	Large salad with ¼ cup of garbanzos. Combine pinto beans, raw broccoli, bean sprouts, shredded carrots, lettuce, and cauliflower.	12	6
Snack	Apple, half pint yogurt.	7	7
Dinner	½ cup soaked brown rice, 1 slice whole-wheat bread, strawberries with milk, 5 oz. baked chicken, or water-pack tuna.	10	30
Snack	Orange, 5 figs, and 2 ozs. of low-fat cheese	5	11
	TOTAL	50	70

Suggested Sensational Substitutes

Negative Risks	Sensational Substitutes
Coffee	Cara-Coa, Instant Carob Drink (El Molino Mills, Industry, CA)
Soft Drinks	Orange juice made with carbonated water is a super delight
	Carbonated apple juice–(Martinelli's Sparkling Apple Juice, Watsonville, CA)
	Pineapple juice with fresh peppermint leaves and ice beaten in blender.

Negative Risks	*Sensational Substitutes*
	Carbonated fruit juice with spices and herbs. No sugar added. (Knudsen & Sons, Chico, CA)
Jello	Pure gelatin with frozen concentrated orange, apple, or grape juice.
Milk Shakes	1 pint plain yogurt put in a blender and mixed with 1 banana and 1 teaspoon rum.
Candy bars	Frozen banana sprinkled with cinnamon or finely chopped English Walnuts.
	Pitted dates with pecan or almond inserted. Roll in finely grated coconut.
	Pineapple slices topped with plain yogurt, then sprinkled with coconut, and lightly frozen.
	Carob coated rice cakes (Chico-San, Inc. Chico, CA 95927)

High Fiber Recipes

CHICKEN CUTLETS SUPREME   5 grams dietary fiber per cutlet
    1 cup Quaker oat bran cereal (uncooked)
    1 tbs. snipped fresh dill or 1 tsp. dried dill weed
    ⅛ tsp lemon pepper
    1 egg
    ¼ cup water
    3 chicken breasts, boned, skinned, and split
    2 tablespoons Butter Buds

Heat oven to 375 F. Spray 13 x 9 inch baking pan with Pam. In shallow dish, combine oat bran cereal, dill and lemon pepper. In another shallow dish, combine egg and water. Lightly pound chicken to even thickness between sheets of plastic wrap or wax paper. Coat with dry ingredients; shake off excess. Dip into egg then coat again with dry ingredients. Place in prepared pan. Drizzle Butter Buds evenly over chicken. Bake 35 minutes. (Serves 6)

STUFFED ZUCCHINI BOATS   7 grams dietary fiber per serving

    4 small zucchini (about 1 lb.)
    1 tbs. Butter Buds
    1 to 2 cloves garlic, minced
    ⅓ cup chopped onion
    1 large tomato, chopped
    1 tsp. dried basil leaves, crushed
    ⅛ tsp. pepper

1 egg
⅔ cup Quaker oat bran cereal, uncooked
½ cup (2 oz.) shredded part-skim Mozzarella cheese

Heat oven to 350F. Spray 13 x 9 inch baking pan with Pam. Place zucchini in large saucepan; add water just tro cover. Simmer 5 to 7 minutes or until tender. Slice lengthwise; hollow out center leaving ¼ inch shell. Chop pulp; reserve.

In medium skillet, melt margarine. Sauté garlic and onion 3 to 4 minutes; add reserved chopped zucchini and tomato. Continue sautéing 2 minutes; remove from heat. Add remaining ingredients except cheese; mix well. Mound mixture evenly into hollowed out zucchini; place in prepared pan. Sprinkle cheese evenly over the zucchini. Bake 35 minutes. (Serves 4)

SEAFOOD SOUFFLE   3 grams dietary fiber per serving

One 15½ oz. can salmon or two 6½ oz. cans water-pack tuna
⅔ cup Quaker oat bran cereal, uncooked
½ cup skimmed milk
¼ cup minced onion
2 tbs. lemon juice
Dash of pepper
1 egg white
2 tbs. minced fresh parsley or 1 tablespoon dried parsley flakes
Dash of paprika

Heat oven to 325 F. Spray 1 qt. glass baking dish or casserole dish with Pam. Drain salmon or tuna; rinse. Remove bones and skin. Separate into large flakes. If using tuna, drain and flake. In large bowl, mix salmon, cereal, milk, onion, lemon juice and pepper. In small mixer bowl, beat egg white at high speed on electric mixer until stiff peaks form; fold into salmon mixture. Pour into prepared dish. Sprinkle with parsley and paprika; bake 45 minutes or until lightly browned. (Serves 6)

CARROT BAKE   4 grams dietary fiber per serving
One 1 lb. package of carrots, shredded
¾ cup Quaker oat bran cereal, uncooked
1 egg
¼ cup water
2 tbs. snipped fresh or frozen chives
2 tbs. chopped nuts
⅛ tsp nutmeg

Heat oven to 350 F. Spray 1 qt. casserole or baking dish with Pam. In large bowl, combine all ingredients. Pour into prepared casserole. Bake 40 minutes. (Serves 8)

TURKEY LOAF WITH CRANBERRY-ORANGE SAUCE   9 grams fiber per serving

1½ lb. uncooked ground turkey
1¼ cups Quaker oat bran cereal, uncooked
½ cup minced onion
½ cup skim or lowfat milk
1 egg
1 tsp. poultry seasoning

Heat oven to 350 F. Spray 9 x 5 inch loaf pan with Pam. In large bowl, combine all ingredients; mix well. Pat into prepared pan. Bake 50-55 minutes. Let stand 5 minutes before slicing. Serve with Cranberry-Orange sauce (recipe follows). (Serves 8)

CRANBERRY-ORANGE SAUCE

2 cups (½ lb.) fresh or frozen cranberries
1¼ cups orange juice
1 tbs. Quaker oat bran cereal, uncooked
1 tsp. fructose sugar (dry)

In medium saucepan, combine all ingredients. Bring to a boil over medium heat. Boil 6 to 7 minutes or until cranberries pop and sauce is thickened. Chill.

EGGPLANT PARMESAN   7 grams fiber per serving

1 medium eggplant (about 1 lb.)
2 medium tomatoes, chopped
one 6 oz. can (⅔ cup) low sodium cocktail vegetable juice
½cup Quaker oat bran cereal, uncooked
1 tsp dried basil leaves, crushed
¼ tsp oregano leaves, crushed
2 cloves garlic, minced
½ cup (2 oz.) part-skim Mozzarella cheese, shredded
2 tablespoons Parmesan cheese

Heat oven to 350 F. Spray 8-inch-square baking dish or 1½ qt. casserole dish with Pam. Peel eggplant; cut into ½ inch slices. Layer into prepared dish; top with tomatoes. In small bowl, combine remaining ingredients except cheeses. Spread over vegetables; sprinkle evenly with Mozzarella cheese, then Parmesan cheese. Bake 35-40 minutes. Serves 4.

CINNAMON OAT BRAN MUFFINS   2 grams dietary fiber per muffin

1¾ cups skim or low-fat milk
1½ cups Quaker oat bran cereal, uncooked

1 egg
⅕ cup fructose (dry)
1 to 1½ tsp. cinnamon
4 tsp. Butter Buds
1 cup whole all-purpose flour (whole grain if possible)
2 tsp. baking powder

Heat oven to 400 F. Spray 12 medium muffin cups with Pam or line with paper baking cups. In medium bowl, combine milk and oat bran cereal. Add egg, fructose, cinnamon and Butter Buds; mix it well. Add combined flour and baking powder to oat bran mixture, mixing just until dry ingredients are moistened. Fill prepared muffin cups ⅔ full. Bake 20 minutes or till light golden brown.

STUFFED TOMATO HALVES   3 grams fiber per tomato half

1 medium green pepper, chopped (about ¾ cup)
4 large tomatoes (about 2 lbs.)
3 to 4 green onions, sliced (about 1 cup)
⅓ cup Quaker oat bran cereal, uncooked
1 egg
¼ to ½ tsp. basil leaves, crushed
¼ to ½ oregano leaves, crushed
2 tbs. chopped fresh parsley or 1 tbs. dried parsley flakes

Heat oven to 350 F. In small saucepan, simmer green pepper in small amount of water 2 to 3 minutes; drain and reserve. Slice each tomato in half crosswise. Scoop out pulp; drain tomato halves upside down. Chop pulp; place in large bowl. Add green pepper and remaining ingredients except parsley. Place tomato halves cut side up in 13½ x 8¾ inch baking dish. Fill each half with about ⅓ cup stuffing mixture; sprinkle parsley over top. Bake about 30 minutes. (Serves 8)

HOT APPLE TREATS   4 grams dietary fiber per cake

2 large corn tortillas or 2 Chico-San rice cakes
Ricotta cheese (Italian skim milk cheese) or cheddar cheese
1 large apple
½ tsp cinnamon

Cut apple into ½ inch slices. Place large corn tortilla on paper plate (if microwaved) or cookie sheet (if oven is used). Lay apple slices in circular fashion on corn tortilla or on the rice cake until top is covered. Grate cheese or lay slices of the cheese on top of the apple slices till barely visible. Sprinkle cinnamon on top as desired. Heat until cheese melts, either in microwave or in broiler. (Serves 2)

COLD APPLE TREATS   2½ grams dietary fiber per cake

Using the same ingredients, substitute apple sauce for the apple to cover the corn tortilla or rice cake. Melt cheese over apple sauce, sprinkle with cinnamon and sandwich with another tortilla or rice cake. Place in freezer 25 minutes to assure semi solid state so that applesauce will not run when chewed.

(Some of these recipes provided courtesy of Quaker Oats Company. For additional high fiber recipes see *The High Fiber Cookbook* by Pamela Westland, Arco Publishing Co., Inc., New York, 1982.)

CHAPTER 6
Selected References

Cheraskin, Emmanuel, and W. M. Ringsdorf. "The Remarkable Homeostatic Effect of a Low Refined Carbohydrate Diet." *Journal of the International Academy of Preventive Medicine,* Vol. IV, No. 1, July 1977, pp. 32–40.

————. *The Vitamin C Connection.* Harper & Row, 1983.

Galton, Lawrence. *The Truth About Fiber in your Food.* Crown Publishing Co., 1976.

Kirby, R. W. et al. "Oat Bran Selectively Lowers Serum Low Density Lipoprotein Cholesterol Concentrations of Hypercholesterolemic Men." *Amer. Journ. Clin. Nutr.,* Vol. 34, 1981.

Strasse-Wolthuis, et. al. "Influence of Dietary Fiber from Vegetables and Fruits, Bran, or Citrus Pectin on Serum Lipids, Fecal Lipids and Colonic Function." *American Journ. Clin. Nutr.,* Vol. 33, 1980, pp. 1745–56.

Van Soest, Peter. "Influence of Dietary Fiber Source on Human Intestinal Transit and Stool Output." *Journ. Nutr.* 113, 1983.

CHAPTER 7

Communication: Beating on Your Chest Won't Work

A Backward Glance

When primitive man developed weapons there occurred a transition from a scavenger of the land to a carnivorous hunter. He became much more predatory. Aggression played a major role in this change because as we became terrestrial there occured a "behavioral transition from retreating to that of an attacking pattern." Thus, aggressive behaviors developed since they had strong survival value.

Also, in order for us to survive (40,000 years ago we lived in bands of 30 to 50 members), fighting within the group had to be avoided. This was accomplished through the development of dominance hierarchies. Aggression played a vital role here also. If a conflict developed, displays of threat by the dominant male (beating on chest, lunging movements, or gruff sounds) were usually sufficient to quiet things down, with the subordinate individual assuming a submissive posture.

Also, as a species, rapid intellectual advancement owes itself to our aggressive nature. The more aggressive, stronger, intelligent males within the dominance hierarchy would mate with the females (polygamy was common) and the weaker males would be less likely to produce offspring. The less intelligent, weaker males were thus selectively eliminated from the gene pool.

The Current Situation

Being a modern animal means being in better control of our aggressive tendencies. To communicate our needs we can no longer jump up and down and beat on our chests as a gesture of threat if we feel slighted or misunderstood. This kind of risk taking is no longer appropriate. Nor is it appropriate to hold things inside passively.

Our modern world is overcrowded and the number of social stressors immense. We must interact with many people, many of whom are total strangers. This makes communication difficult.

Our businesses and corporations certainly have dominance hierarchies (the "executive ladder") and aggression, being part of our heritage, can certainly explode. But the important thing to remember, as studies on aggression have shown, is that the aggression depends on events in the social environment. This is the trigger. You will learn how to defuse this trigger.

Whether at home or work, aggression rarely serves a constructive purpose. As a modern animal we need to develop a more sophisticated approach to communicate our feelings and our needs. This is best accomplished with the active listening and assertiveness, two wellness skills that have broad implications. By learning to interact more effectively with others, you accomplish three things. You:

1. Create a wellness challenge that can lead to new growth (positive risk taking).
2. Create a more stimulating lifestyle. People are exciting sources of stimulation.
3. Learn to be more assertive. This wellness skill will help you manage your stresses much better.

Measuring Current Life Stresses

Before you learn these skills, you ought to measure your current life stresses. Much of what you learn will apply toward reducing those that produce distress.

In the following list, check off every item which refers to something going on in your life right now. Don't borrow trouble, but ask the question, "Does this apply to me and my life right now?" This stress survey was developed by Dr. Gerald Sheridan, a psychologist at the University of Missouri at Kansas City.

1. Dealing with my children's problems and questions.
2. Rarely or never having too much to do.
3. Feeling accepted by others.
4. Experiencing high level noise at work or home.
5. Having my mother or father say something like: "You don't really love me."
6. Being clear about what is expected of me.
7. Planning an important contract or piece of work.
8. Demanding my rights at work.
9. Feeling I have no real purpose in life.
10. Having someone call something I've done "stupid."

11. Having my leisure plans upset.
12. Feeling committed at home or at work.
13. Not having to cope with bureaucratic machinery.
14. Having my primary-relationship partner (spouse or mate) stare at a possible rival who seems quite attractive.
15. Not going along with the group.
16. Seeing little challenge in my work or play.
17. Asserting my rights or privileges.
18. Watching or reading the news.
19. Having someone act as if they dislike me.
20. Having my sexual needs met.
21. Being around angry people.
22. Being watched while I'm working.
23. Suffering a loss of status.
24. Having things to do that interest me.
25. Working or living in situations where things are well organized.
26. Watching an argument between members of my family.
27. Having regular opportunities to express my viewpoint.
28. Getting to have a good laugh.
29. Giving a speech before a group of relative strangers.
30. Having little control over what happens to me.
31. Making decisions that affect my family's future.
32. Carrying out work that is mentally demanding.
33. Rarely or never suffering from discomfort or pain.
34. Finding myself in a position in my primary relationship where anything I say or do will be wrong.
35. Making major decisions in my life.
36. Being around people who are talking in a loud voice.
37. Rarely or never working against a tight deadline.
38. Experiencing a great deal of family friction.
39. Feeling angry.
40. Rarely or never traveling on congested public transport or in traffic jams.
41. Failing or forgetting to perform some important responsibility.
42. Living a stimulating, interesting life.
43. Keeping my emotions to myself.
44. Having opportunities to have fun.
45. Making decisions independently.
46. Being interviewed for a job.
47. Having my abilities at work valued and put to good use.
48. Being bombarded by questions and requests.
49. Having sleep patterns that are good and regular.
50. Having the authority to meet my responsibilities at work.
51. Having enough time to myself.
52. Thinking about major problems confronting me.

53. Angrily telling someone off.
54. Knowing the end product of my work.
55. Having variation or fresh stimulation in my sexual activities.
56. Losing my health and being forced to change my lifestyle.
57. Being able to perform statisfactorily on my job.
58. Having to make decisions where I will lose out no matter what I do.
59. Spending time in work areas or rooms that are drab, uncomfortable, and depressing.
60. Being in a situation where I am unsure of the right thing to do.
61. Having thoughts of losing my primary-relationship partner or someone else dear to me.
62. Having enough money to meet expenses.
63. Moving away from home to a new town.
64. Losing my job.
65. Having a nourishing well-balanced diet.
66. Getting enough exercise.
67. Having to do jobs I can't cope with.
68. Rarely or never having to do jobs I have no interest in.
69. Getting the rewards I had hoped for.
70. Having a low opinion of myself.
71. Rarely or never working long hours.
72. Having enough leisure time.
73. Being overburdened with responsibility.
74. Having the opportunity to see friends socially.
75. Undergoing disruption of my marriage.
76. Rarely or never having to work at jobs that are too simple for me.
77. Working at a task that requires constant attention, but leaves little room for initiative.
78. Having to work with inadequate lighting.
79. Feeling that something extremely unpleasant could happen to me or to someone close to me and being helpless to do anything about it.
80. Feeling I have friends or relatives who will help me when I need help.

Scoring

A. For each item with a SHADED number you did not check, add a point to your score. Write in your total number of points here._____

B. Now, count the number of items you checked that are NOT SHADED. For each of these items, add one to your score. Then write in the total points from uncircled items here._____

C. Add point totals for A and B above to get your stress rating score._____

If your score is close to 35, you have an average level of stress in your life. But remember, the average stress level in our society is quite high.

If your score includes as many as 45 items, you are notably higher on stressors than the average person. You need to digest and implement information in this chapter and in the book itself.

A score of 55 or more is very high. It is critical to your wellness that you learn to relax (see chapter 12) and implement the nutrition and exercise recommendations. Understanding this chapter will measurably improve your relationships with others.

Some test items dealt with too much or too little stimulation. This is a topic we will discuss at length later on.

Develop Active Listening Skills

Now, look at your stress survey. Note how often questions dealt with social stressors. At least half of the test items (those involving people and situations) could be improved through developing good communication skills. This is an essential part of wellness and stress management. For example, Dr. James Lynch, at the University of Maryland Medical School, has found that talking increases systolic blood pressure. Those who suffer from high blood pressure and/or talk very fast are at higher risk because the systolic blood pressure can increase dramatically. By learning to speak more slowly, breathe more regularly, and listen (really listen), a person can cause his or her own blood pressure to return to normal.

Try this experiment: Next time someone yells in anger or disgust within your presence, instead of getting excited, remain calm and simply respond by saying, "You sound angry (disgusted, disappointed, etc.) (Name) Are you just angry or are you angry at me?" If your angry person is relatively sane, they should answer something like this, "No, I'm not angry at you, I'm just angry because _____(I lost something, hate this job, am tired, etc.).

Let me introduce you to one of the simplest yet most effective tools for high-level wellness—active listening. It is an extremely effective tool that controls stress in the following ways:

First, by acknowledging the other person's anger, you defuse a potential explosion. Anger held inside is a "negative risk."

Second, it answers the question "to whom was the anger directed?" Is it anger directed toward you the listener, toward some inanimate object, or some other person?

Third, it buys time for you to analyze the nature of the anger so you don't get caught up in the storm. You have recognized the other person's frustration or anger and yet have objectively removed yourself from participating in the situation. You can remain calm. You can gather additional information before forming your own opinion on the situation.

There are three processes to communication, the person who sent the message (the speaker), the receiver of the message (the responder), and the content contained in the message. Such messages may be verbal or nonverbal (body language, written messages, etc.).

Dis-stress results when one or more of the three processes is inadequate, incomplete, or distorted in some way. Misunderstanding then occurs, and emotions can get out of hand.

For example, someone you work with blurts out, "I hate this job!" You feel yourself aroused by this aggressive display and take the comment personally. Then you think, "What did I do? Why are they angry at me?" instead of removing yourself from the remark and questioning such assumptions as not directed at you. Active listening can cut this emotional chain. Active listening means keeping your poise when all around you seems chaotic, confused, or otherwise intense. Very often the responder only acts to heighten the intensity with remarks like, "I know, it's a rotten job, I can't stand it either." Such a response only fuels the flame rather than suffocating it. Think about why you might tend to respond this way. Perhaps you think this will calm the other person or direct the anger away from you. It doesn't. Sometimes people just want to let off steam, especially if they don't have a physical outlet as we discussed in chapter 5.

An alternative response, based upon active listening and sensitivity to the angry person's feelings, might go like this:

SPEAKER: "I hate this job!"

RESPONDER: "Well, you sound pretty upset."

SPEAKER: "Sure, wouldn't you, they hire someone new in the department and pay them about the same as me and I've been here two years."

RESPONDER: I'm sorry you're upset. I wanted to see if you were mad at me for some reason or just upset about the job."

However the conversation goes after this, several things have resulted from the active listening approach.

1. Emotions have been cooled, both the speaker's and the listener's.
2. The delayed response of the listener has allowed time to analyze the nature of the remark in terms of implied feelings or emotions.
3. The listener is better able to control the flow of conversation thereafter because the speaker has sensed concern from the other person.

I want to provide some guidelines to follow in this technique of active listening. I am indebted to Dr. Jenny Steinmetz, a psychologist at the University of California Medical Center in San Diego, for categorizing the pitfalls that can occur.

Avoid "fueling the fire" when someone makes an emotionally charged statement. For example, If someone blurts out, "I should've been promoted a year ago!" how would you respond? Do you say something like "Yeah, you really should have, this place is so unfair." *No.* This verifies nothing, but only adds to the intensity of emotion expressed.

Avoid defensive reactions on your part. Example: Your spouse (girlfriend, etc.) says something like, "You told me we were going to dinner tonight and now you come home and tell me your brother is coming over here for dinner!" A defensive response might go something like this; "Well, we can always go out to dinner but my brother doesn't get in town that often!" Once again, the stress level has only been escalated and the stage is set for a heated debate. No feelings are resolved.

Avoid making a "judgment call" by placing your own interpretation on the motive, emotion, or personality of the person who's upset. For example, if someone blurts out "Everytime I open up my feelings to someone I get hurt!" A judgment call might go something like this: "That's because you have such a low opinion of yourself and you're just hungry for love." All you've done is play psychologist or minimized the importance of the message when you really needed to be an "active listener."

Avoid "lending a helping hand" by supporting the statement. This is difficult to avoid because it is part of our nature to be helping others. For example, Someone complains: "A lot of people around here take 20- or 25-minute breaks and get away with it." You respond: "I know, I understand, don't worry, I'll help you get through this." The basis for the emotional outpouring never got resolved and you've waded in knee-deep. Are you prepared to assume the burden for the problem?

Avoid "mimicking," where you matter-of-factly restate the other person's message. For example, someone says, "My husband (wife, boyfriend, etc.) is so selfish!" To this you respond "Sounds like your husband is really selfish." This kind of response is a total putdown of the other person as unimportant and insignificant. You were nothing more than a parrot. You failed to acknowledge the intent of the message.

Active listening is the most effective way of responding to someone who is angry, upset, or otherwise aroused. It allows you to act as a mirror to the upset person. Some other possible responses are listed below.

"You _____ sound _____	hurt _____	about _____ this."
seem	worried	them.
appear	discouraged	that.
	disturbed	

A final example of this listening technique follows:

SPEAKER: "I'm so hurt. I wish he/she could accept me exactly the way I am without trying to change me all the time."

ACTIVE LISTENER: "You sound like you can't quite understand why he treated you that way."

I should warn you of something many of us may unconsciously do from time to time. This is to *CREATE* high stimulation by "fueling the fire" when we detect excitement in someone else. We may do this for the arousal it provides without realizing the impact it can have on the other person. This may be especially true for those people who have high sensation-seeking needs, as we will see later in the book. This is a sick way to counteract a boring life, at someone else's expense. If you find yourself doing this, then something is drastically wrong and I hope you thoroughly digest chapters 14 and 15. You may also wish to read Dr. Lynche's book *Language of the Heart—The Body's Response to Human Dialogue* (Basic Books, 1985).

Active listening should not be a facade, an artificial way of humoring the other person. It should arise from four qualities:

1. A genuine concern for people.
2. A sense of equality for everyone—"Everyone has a right to voice their feelings."
3. An understanding and acceptance of problems and difficulties as part of life.
4. A desire for personal growth through effective interaction with others.

Active listening tends to relax the aroused person so they can continue to express their emotions and begin the problem solving process. By avoiding the five pitfalls discussed earlier you'll avoid adding to an already charged situation. Try to be aware of this technique more often, practice it and you will become a more sensitive individual. It promotes behavioral changes conducive to high-level wellness and peak performance.

Learn to be Assertive

Look back at the Sheridan stress survey you filled out earlier in this chapter. See if you checked numbers 8, 10, 17, 21, 36, 39, 43, 48, 53, 73 and 78. These are all social stressors that arise from interactions with others. Typically, we develop a lot of stress because we either hold in our feelings or blurt them out inappropriately. Clearly we need a way to state our feelings in a diplomatic way.

The first step in the process, active listening, helps you to recognize what the other person is experiencing. With assertiveness training, you get to express yourself.

The important thing to remember in being assertive is that you are getting your feelings out so anger, guilt, or fear doesn't build up, while not downgrading someone else. The difference between "you're wrong" and

"I don't agree with you" is that in the second statement you have not attacked the other person's self-esteem.

An example will help here. I used to lend books from my health library. More often than not they didn't get returned so I'd get angry, upset, and just plain mad when I had to go calling people to return them. This caused me a lot of distress. Now when someone asks to borrow a book I simply say, "I'm sorry, I make it a policy never to loan books out. You're perfectly welcome to come by anytime and look them over here." This is a lot better than saying, "No, you can't borrow it; you won't bring it back." This last remark is an assault on the other person's integrity. People simply forget. Handling it in an assertive way keeps both of us from being overstressed.

Isn't it frustrating when we want to make our needs known, let people know when something bothers us at home or work? We want to make our needs or interests known, but do it in a style which is (1) effective, (2) pleasant, and (3) controlled. Yelling doesn't meet these criteria. Beating on your chest might work temporarily, but the next day when you show up for work, there will probably be some men in white uniforms waiting to take you away. Being nice with the idea that somehow others will interpret your needs doesn't meet these criteria either. (The medical aspects of this are discussed in Chapter 14.)

Let's now list some other characteristics of assertiveness.

1. Assertiveness is *assuming responsibility* for your own emotions rather than letting someone else assume ownership.
2. It is *phrasing things* in such a way that people will listen and will feel relaxed about responding.
3. It is, more than anything else, *honesty.* You act and react in a direct self-respecting, self-expressing, and straight-forward manner.
4. It is *goal oriented,* designed to achieve good two way interaction between people. This leaves both people feeling good about themselves which controls stress and enhances self-esteem.

Passive Versus Aggressive Behavior Styles

Before we can put this technique into practice, we need to differentiate it from two extreme forms of behavior that create distress: aggressive and passive behavior. Let me define them.

Passive behavior means we allow other people to choose for us. We play the martyr because we practice self-denial. This mode of behavior is emotionally dishonest and can be like a time bomb. In denying our own rights we silently "keep score" of all the things or people which caused anger (and hostility) but never got expressed.

For example, you want to be the "perfect spouse." So, when you are asked to run an errand to the store you do so. When you are asked to get the phone and take some messages while your partner watches a TV program you say, "Sure, okay," even though you were watching the same program with the same keen interest. Then, when your spouse gets ready for bed and says "Honey, will you feed the dog," you yell, "No! Feed the damn dog yourself!"

The anger built up. You thought you were in control, when in fact you were being controlled by merit of your passive behavior. Inside you were saying to yourself, "It isn't fair," but those feelings never got expressed properly.

Occasionally, being passive may work if you simply desire no interaction, but this is usually not the case. The passive person needs to relinquish the false notion that, "I don't have a right to make myself known, to make others feel uncomfortable or displeased." This attitude is closely tied to a low self-concept. Asserting your needs can be the first step to enhancing your self-concept. In effect you are saying, "I am a worthwhile and important person. I want others to know my feelings, attitudes and ideas about the world."

Dr. Harry Jordan, a psychiatrist at the University of Pennsylvania and author of *The Doctor's Calories-Plus Diet,* found in his research that being assertive rather than passive was a key factor in successfully maintaining weight reduction. He states: "Assertiveness is necessary because it helps control one's life."

Aggression is the other extreme. Aggressive people have a high need to control not only themselves but everyone else also. These people tend to be extremely self-centered and honest in a socially unacceptable way. They make their feelings known in a very tactless way. The aggressive communicator achieves the goal, establishes his or her needs, but at your expense. You get put down if you are at the receiving end. In upholding *your* rights you are often made to feel humiliated, defensive, resentful, and hurt.

Try to avoid these kinds of people if possible. If you have to work with someone like this it can be very stressful indeed. For example: "You don't get things done fast enough to suit me. You better speed things up."

This statement immediately puts you down and humiliates you.

Risk Taking

As I will point out in later chapters, being assertive is a form of social risk taking. You are always faced with options or choices of how to respond. You can be passive, aggressive, or assertive. The first two are negative risks because they cause long-term stress, which is very harmful (see chapter 9). Being assertive, on the other hand, is a positive risk that can enhance communication and self-confidence. Even here, however, you need to know when the "positive risk" is warranted. Speaking out, even assertively, may cost you your job, your lover, or some other attachment—a relative or friend. It is social risk taking and you have to decide which option you want.

Several weeks ago I attended a movie that was really packed. Just before the movie began I saw a couple move down the aisle in front of me. The man asked the two women already seated in front of us if they would move down a seat so there would be two adjoining seats. One woman assertively said, "No, I don't want to move." She could have been very aggressive and said "You don't have any right to barge in here and try to make us move." Instead, she was assertive. But her companion convinced her it wouldn't matter if they moved one seat down. In this case, being passive would probably have sufficed. It was more realistic to just move, especially since it didn't affect their view of the screen, and the inconvenience was minor. One can carry assertiveness to extremes. Use good judgment.

Comparison of Alternative Behavior Styles

Now look at the accompanying chart on page 104 and circle the items that best describe you. Then you'll know how often you are assertive, aggressive, or passive.

How do assertive people act?

They establish *direct eye contact*. This reflects their desire to establish good communication. It doesn't mean they try to stare other people down, they simply want good two way understanding.

They often use your *first name* since informality is often a prelude to a more open, honest conversation. Of course, there are times when formality is necessary. Even then you may cut the ice by asking the other person to use your first name.

They may use *hand gestures,* an effective way of emphasizing the content and importance of your message. This doesn't mean act as if you're directing traffic but, rather, emphasizing your point.

Other techniques include *good posture*, strong, clear, crisp *speaking voice*. The tone of your voice alone can convey different messages even if the same words are used. When being assertive, don't end a statement with your voice trailing off as though you are seeking approval. For example, "I want some time to myself this afternoon, okay . . ?" Be firm to let the other person know the matter is closed. Being assertive means knowing when to stop talking. To use the same example, "I am going to take some time for myself this afternoon."

Try to *make "I" statements* rather than "you" statements. This establishes *your* needs. For example, one of the hardest things to do is say no when asked to do something we really don't want to do.

Let's examine two alternative ways of responding to the question, "Will you take me to the movies?"

	Passive	Assertive	Aggressive
Characteristics	Allow others to choose for you. Emotionally dishonest. Indirect, self-denying, inhibited. In win-lose situations you lose. If you do get your own way, it is indirect.	Choose for self. Appropriately honest. Direct, self-respecting, self-expressing, straightforward. Convert win-lose to win-win.	Choose for others. Inappropriately honest (tactless). Direct, self-enhancing. Self-expressive, derogatory. Win-lose situation which you win.
Your own feelings on the exchange	Anxious, ignored, helpless, manipulated. Angry at yourself and/or others.	Confident, self-respecting, goal oriented, valued. Later: accomplished.	Righteous, superior, depreciatory, controlling. Later: possibly guilty.
Others' feelings in the exchange	Guilty or superior. Frustrated with you.	Valued, respected.	Humiliated, defensive, resentful, hurt.
Others' view of you in the exchange	Lack of respect. Distrust. Can be considered a pushover. Do not know where you stand.	Respect, trust, know where you stand.	Vengeful, angry, distrustful, fearful.
Outcome	Others achieve their goals at your expense. Your rights are violated.	Outcome determined by above-board negotiation. Your and others' rights respected.	You achieve your goal at others' expense. Your rights upheld; others violated.
Underlying belief system	I should never make anyone uncomfortable or displeased . . . except myself.	I have a responsibility to protect my own rights: I respect others but not necessarily their behavior.	I have to put others down to protect myself.

1. "Don't you want me to have some time to myself?"
2. "No, I need some time to myself."

In the first alternative you project a sense of guilt if you say no. You're shirking your responsibility for your deeper feelings. In the second, you are taking responsibility for your own decision making.

This example points out a common myth you want to avoid. It goes like this: "If I tell you what I need, you're going to feel obligated to do it." Again, this is shifting *your* responsibility to the other person.

Assertive people also *keep sentences short*. Long, windy, rambling statements project a fear of disapproval.

Practice these skills whenever possible. Remember, in high-level wellness there are no failures, only nonsuccesses. As you try out your new assertiveness skills you'll feel a real sense of accomplishment as you become better able to make your needs known. You may also help ward off some disease. One research study found that extroverted people (those who openly express their needs and feelings), were more healthy and less susceptible to heart disease and cancer. Nevertheless, various aspects of human behavior, which communication certainly is, do not exist in a vacuum. Everything interrelates. As you eat better, exercise more, visualize your goals, and learn to relax, you'll grow more confident in every way. Then, you'll be more able to assert yourself.

If, after considerable practice, you continue to experience anxiety and fear about being assertive with someone in your life, such as your spouse or employer, then read the next section and learn how to desensitize yourself to fear.

Systematic Desensitization

A technique often used in clinical psychology to reduce anxiety and fear is called *systematic desensitization*. It is the same technique I used to manage the fears associated with my stunts. It simply means gradually exposing oneself to more intense levels of the fear while learning to relax and practice a new skill such as assertiveness.

The usual problem is this: We have great difficulty expressing our true feelings to the people we're closest to, whereas we can easily do so with those we have no emotional ties to. But, the irony of it is that the people we are closest to are the ones we get affection, attention, approval, and acceptance from. This is exactly why we need to communicate effectively with them.

Let's now examine how the procedure works. First, sit down and make a list of those you want to be more assertive with. Beside each person write down a situation requiring assertiveness which causes you anxiety. Some examples are indicated below.

People	Situations
Others	Merely asserting my rights
Store clerks	Asserting my own preferences
Salesmen and solicitors	Saying "NO", not interested
Angry customers	Defending our policies
In-laws	Requesting privacy
Friends	Communicating expectations
Children	Can't say "no" to requests
Co-workers	Not assuming job roles
Immediate supervisor	Demanding my rights
Husband or boyfriend	Differences of opinion

List some real situations in your life where assertiveness could help. Try to place them in order of priority, with the one that causes the least anxiety on top and the one that causes the most anxiety on the bottom.

Start at the top with situations where assertion is easy, and continue to practice more often, letting others know where you stand. As you work down the list you will reach a point where, despite your best intentions, you may revert to your aggressive or passive method of reacting. If this is the case, return to the technique discussed in Chapter 4. Imagine yourself asserting your true feelings. Use visualization with deep breathing to achieve a deep state of relaxation. By combining your visual imagery with actual successes you will reap the greatest returns, because your images will probably be more vivid.

Once you learn to express your needs more effectively, your relationships will improve. Family, friends, and others will respect you more, you'll be on your way toward peak performance.

CHAPTER 7
Selected References

Steinmetz, Jenny et al. *Managing Stress Before It Manages You.* Bull Publishing, 1980.

CHAPTER 8

Relaxation: Be Your Own Witch Doctor

A Backward Glance

Even our primitive ancestors had to devise ways of managing stress. How did they do this? Through religion? All religions rest upon a belief in the supernatural. But to tap into the supernatural power source they needed a "chosen one," who had access to gods and spirits beyond that of ordinary men.

Enter the shaman. No anthropologist has yet penetrated to a tribe so primitive that it does not have shamans. Let me describe this devious rascal.

Some degree of emotional instability was an essential trait of the shaman, who obtained his position by mystical experience (although some inherited the position). He or she had to be capable of hallucinations. Modern psychiatry would most certainly have labeled these unstable individuals "schizophrenic." To be a spirit-endowed shaman the odds favored those who belonged to the "lunatic fringe." Their magic skills were impressive. Ventriloquism was a favored tool; by shifting voices around they appeared able to control the spirit world. They were also quite exploitative at times, with male shamans taking advantage of married and unmarried women to gratify themselves sexually in the name of the gods. Some would hold impressive seances while secretly manipulating the tent so it would rock and pitch violently with the arrival of a spirit.

Still, a positive social service was provided, for the shaman gave the tribe members a feeling of control over life's uncertain events. In a collective sense they were more relaxed.

The Current Situation

The shaman is gone, but only in name. The "shamen" of today are the pill promoters with their arsenal of pain relievers, muscle relaxants, tran-

107

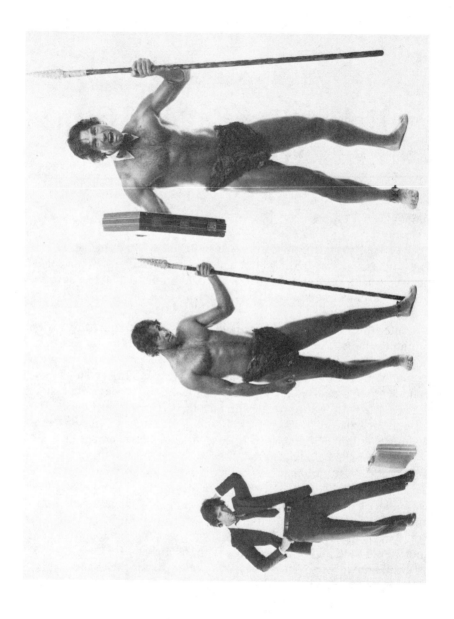

quilizers, and antidepressants. Indeed, they define depression as a "valium deficiency."

These people know full well how stressed, tense, and fatigued most of you are and they spend literally millions to convince you they have the answer to what ails you. Of course the question arises, how did we ever exist without these various pharmacological agents? Truth is, we didn't need them except on very rare occasions. We felt in control for the most part.

We have come a long way since our primitive times. Our superior knowledge has given us much more understanding of life and its events. Still, as Homo sapiens we have been catapulted in one quantum leap into an age of space travel and mass communication at an incredible rate. Many of us are confused, for our brains and nervous system were never designed to handle such large sensory inputs of information. Lost, we wander among the skyscrapers, enclosed in our steel chariots, weaving our way through the maze of neon lights, billboards, and stoplights, looking for the right direction.

Because the pace is so fast, we need to stop and pause, to unwind, to give our brain and nervous systems some respite from the massive sensory overload we are faced with in today's world. There's a general consensus among mental health professionals that a lot of substance abuse, use of medications (tranquilizers, pain relievers, antidepressants, etc.) are caused by an inability to manage the daily pressures we encounter.

Of course, the drug industry spends millions on TV ads to convince you that pharmacological agents are the appropriate way to resolve tension in your life. After all, it does look convincing when that old steel worker takes an Anacin and walks across that high beam hundreds of feet above the ground with no more headaches, right? How about Grandma? If she hadn't had that pain reliever those kids who jumped in her lap would've gotten their britches warmed, right? Next time you have your car worked on be sure and give the mechanic some Rolaids (as you smile lovingly). He'll fix your car in half the time and your bill will be less, right? Wrong. The old steel worker developed ulcers to replace his headache and took early retirement; Grandma finally slapped one of the little urchins when the pain reliever wore off and was promptly sent to the old folks' home; and the mechanic (suspecting you jimmied with the pills) threw the Rolaids in the trash and charged you more anyway. Yes, the shamans are still here, they've just changed their wardrobes.

Stress Management Techniques

Having been involved in stress management programs for nine years now, I've seen a lot of confused people who can't make heads or tails out of all the hokus pokus, mumbo-jumbo, razzamatazz and other claims on how to manage stress. So, before telling you what I consider to be the best way to learn how to relax, let me list the techniques used in stress management programs and give a brief description of how each one can help turn stress into a positive force so we can function at peak performance.

Stress Management Techniques

Physical: Improve stress tolerance
     Methods: Exercise
                Nutrition
                Adequate sleep
Cognitive: Remove stresses
     Methods: Rationalization (much of our self-talk is self-defeating, not based on rational analysis of the actual facts)
                Make major life changes as necessary
                Examine values and goals
                Alter harmful behavior traits
Holistic: Alter stress response (fight or flight)
     Methods: Meditation
                Visualization (guided imagery)
                Progressive muscle relaxation
                Hypnosis
                Isolation tank
                Biofeedback training
                Desensitization training
                Deep-breathing methods
                Music therapy
                Prayer
Pharmacologic: Medical (last resort or in times of crisis)
     Methods: Sedatives
                Tranquilizers
                Anti-depressants
                Beta blockers

The *physical* methods increase your energy levels and general resistance and thus improve your stress tolerance. An engineer who designs a bridge calculates the forces (weight, number of cars at any time, etc.) in order to compute how much concrete and support rods are needed. I've already discussed exercise and nutrition in this regard: when we maximize those factors we have, in effect, added more concrete and strengthened our pillars so we can handle greater loads. Of course, sleep is important to restore us and the quality of sleep is highly dependent upon knowing how and when to go hard (exercise) and how and when to let go (relax).

Cognitive methods function primarily by eliminating the unwanted sources of stress (*dis*-stress), which is like reducing the number of cars on the bridge to reduce the weight factor. It is in this area that a trained counselor can help you determine whether certain life changes (divorce, changing jobs, etc.) are the answer or to learn to view things objectively rather than be a victim of your emotional reactions and negative self-talk. Chapter 7 dealt with some of this—learning to make your needs known— and other portions of the book touch on examination of values.

I've already mentioned the *pharmacologic* approach and should add two points. First, there are rare times when, because of a major life crisis, this approach is warranted. Pharmacological agents have their place but keep in mind that, according to statistics gathered by the National Wellness Center, over 80 percent of the visits to physicians are due to depression, boredom, unhappiness, and general discontent with life rather than some medical emergency or crisis. Second, when people won't take responsibility for themselves, then pharmacological agents are better than nothing. My real concern is the people who abuse drugs in attempts to cope with life or simply use them for stimulation seeking. For example, a survey at the University of Colorado showed that 96 percent of the student body used alcohol regularly, 49 percent smoked marijuana regularly, and 36 percent used cocaine regularly. There are many natural ways to get a "Rocky Mountain high." I'll describe one shortly.

Finally, we have the *holistic* approach, so-called because it's something we can do ourselves in most cases and because it is designed to help us regain mind/body balance in numerous ways. The goal is to alter the stress response, changing our perception of the event so we interpret it in a positive fashion. What we do is disengage the sudden response of the hypothalamus, a gland at the base of the brain that mediates the alarm reaction and triggers the release of potentially dangerous hormones like adrenalin. By controlling how we interpret an event—a reaction that happens at the cerebral cortex or outer half-inch of the brain—we can alter the response of the hypothalamus and handle the same event with more composure, if not total control. To use the bridge analogy again, this is like making lighters cars to go over the bridge, thus reducing the effect of each car (event).

I've trained people in each of these various stress techniques at hospitals, corporations, or other wellness facilities for some ten years. What I've seen has been largely disappointing.

Most of these techniques are basically sound; that is, they *do* alter the stress response but if, *and only if,* a substantial training program is followed for a certain number of weeks and the person maintains the structure by regular attendance to master the skills involved. Of course, some methods are learned more quickly than others. However, ongoing programs are rare. Most stress management programs focus upon introducing people to progressive muscle relaxation, biofeedback, or deep breathing methods with little regard to whether such skills have been learned sufficiently to aid the user in specific situations of distress. As one man put it, "Great, I can sit here and get real relaxed, but when I go out the front door, the tensions are still there. Nothing's changed."

For relaxation to be truly effective we need a technique that:

1. Can be learned quickly.
2. Requires as little effort as possible on the part of the individual who desires it (this is the lure of drugs).
3. Has effects that are long lasting, that carry over to life outside the learning environment.

The Flotation Tank

This brings us to the *flotation tank,* a modern version of the tank developed by Dr. John Lilly some 30 years ago for the purpose of studying restricted environmental stimulation. Dr. Lilly believed there were worlds of experience that went beyond the five senses, frontiers to be explored once free of our body's normal gravitational field and states of consciousness most people never probe. But probe them he did. His research made him famous and opened up a whole new dimension in the study of behavior and relaxation.

The flotation tank is both mystical and scientific, creative yet reproducible in its effects. To attempt to describe its many uses and implications, medical and otherwise in one chapter is a challenge in itself.

The flotation tank is a soundproof, lightproof chamber filled with about 10 or 12 inches of saltwater. This saltwater is carefully maintained at 93.5° F (normal skin temperature) to eliminate the tactile (touch) sense. The flotation tank thus effectively filters out most of the stimulation that bombards our brain, not the least of which is gravity. It's been estimated by physiologists that 85 percent of our energy is expended to offset the effects of gravity. Because of the extremely high salt content (27 percent) of the flotation tank, a near-zero-gravity environment—weightlessness—is produced. In this environment it is very easy to let go completely, to free the mind from its space-time reference points and from intense activation of sensory input; to let it wander and experience a "psychological free-fall."

What usually happens then is a gradual progression from asynchronous brain wave activity called beta to alpha and in many cases, even theta brain waves. This progression is depicted on page 113.

The progression reflects a state of altered consciousness from an excited state of electrical brainwave activity (beta) to one indicative of meditation (alpha or theta). At that point, as shown, all the neurons (nerves) are firing in synchrony and, if recorded on an electroencephalograph (EEG), the high-amplitude, low-frequency theta waves would be seen. This deep state of relaxation is what people who learn to meditate try to achieve. Once there, anything goes. In many cases people report sudden resolution of problems, great insights of creative thinking, out-of-body experiences, and what may generally be called a re-centering of

Brainwave Activity

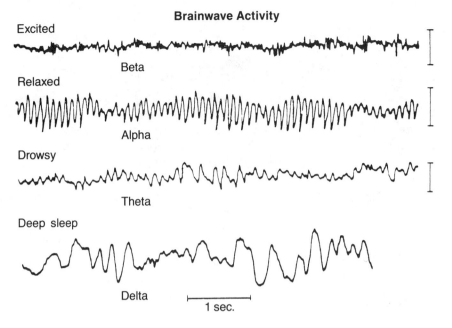

Excited

Beta

Relaxed

Alpha

Drowsy

Theta

Deep sleep

Delta

1 sec.

oneself, a feeling of having gained control over their life and feeling potent once again.

Scientific Basis for Flotation

Is there any scientific basis or support for such reports? Indeed there is. Much of the research in this area has been supported by grants from Float to Relax in Lakewood, Colorado, in order to examine the subjective claims. In one of these studies, Dr. Gary Stern at the University of Colorado demonstrated an increase in theta brainwave activity (8-12 cycles/sec) indicative of deep relaxation; decreases in EMG activity of the muscles, indicating the occurrence of a tranquilizer-like effect; and positive mood changes as the result of using the float tank. As of this writing, 20 major universities have/or are studying the effects of Restricted Environmental Stimulation Tanks (R.E.S.T.).

Some of the data has shown improved problem-solving ability and improved retention of learned material while in the tank. Dr. Thomas Taylor of College Station, Texas, tested two groups of students. Some students floated while being presented several different concepts; a control group listened to the same material while lying on a couch in quiet, dark room. Students who floated were able to synthesize (interrelate) the material better than a control group that was presented the same raw information:

The results show that the more difficult the concept, the bigger the difference in the performance of the two groups . . . the only difference in the two groups was that the experimental group was floating.

Additional findings include lowered oxygen consumption, enhancement of the immune system (which could prevent disease caused by bacterial and viral microorganisms), and reductions in chronic pain for patients suffering from arthritis.

Purely as a mode of stimulation and pleasure alone, the research indicates flotation can be effective. Neuroendocrinologist John Turner, at the Medical College of Ohio, using double-blind procedures to ensure strict control and validity of findings, found that floating in sensory-restricted tanks caused the release of beta-endorphins, natural opiates of the body which block pain sensations, to produce mood states of euphoria and well-being. Perhaps this is why use of the flotation tanks has proven highly effective in lowering blood pressure and helping people to lose weight, stop smoking, decrease alcohol consumption, and generally manage stress better.

Transcendence with Flotation

Although the scientific validation is there, the mystical/spiritual experience is no less in terms of relaxation of body, mind, and soul. What typically happens is a kind of transcendence wherein the person feels more in touch with the spiritual self, as though a cleansing process has occurred. This may be similar to the *peak experience* described by Dr. Abraham Maslow, a famous psychologist. Maslow wrote in *Religions, Values and Peak Experiences* that while transcendence of self is a very natural thing, it provides us with greater illumination or revelation of our relationship to the rest of the world. This does not mean supernatural, but rather a totally private and personal experience after which the "peaker" discovers, develops, and retains a greater understanding of self and purpose. Dr. Maslow often referred to this as "developing an X-ray texture of the world," that is, being able to see beneath the surface of other people, places, things, and feeling a greater sense of truth.

Each person adds his own unique interpretation to the float experience just as everyone who views an impressionistic painting finds something personal in the images. To experience sharper senses, to see colors more vividly, or touch or smell the world as a child discovering things for the first time is to be more alive. Many people report a feeling of greater love in that they become more spontaneous, honest, and innocent. For others, time becomes less a God, and the dichotomies, polarities, and conflicts of life seem transcended. People calm down.

How long do these effects last? Is one forever bound to a float tank? The "wash-out" period in one study was found to be about three weeks. The cost of floating for one hour is about $20.00 or less. The cost of traditional medical therapy for some of the conditions mentioned costs considerably more and carries the risk of adverse side effects. Isn't depression a valium deficiency? The statistics lead us to think so, when close to 50 million prescriptions were sold last year. Valium is taken by over 20 million Americans. Between 1976 and 1977, some 54,400 people sought emergency room treatment for problems caused by excess Valium consumption, and 17,600 people sought emergency room treatment for taking too much aspirin. No one has ever required emergency room treatment for an hour of floating. I doubt they ever will, even though thousands of people float daily.

Flotation Uses with Other Modalities

The beautiful thing about floating is that it can be supplemented with all other holistic modalities listed. Meditation (not to be confused with transcendental meditation or TM) as described by Dr. Herbert Benson in *The Relaxation Response* can be used when not in the tank to produce some (but not all) of the same results, although as indicated earlier most people fail to expend the time and energy to maintain this skill. If you can't float, meditation via the relaxation response is the next best thing.

I always used the relaxation response before one of my fearful adventures to calm myself and control anxiety. Studies have shown it reduces the buildup of lactic acid, which can trigger anxiety attacks. But, like other meditators who eventually slack off, I'd stop doing it, only to force myself back into the routine when things became too stressful. I only wish I'd had R.E.S.T. available then (as now) because it's so easy to meditate while floating. For those who wish to learn meditation the easy way the tank is the perfect aid. For example, Dr. John Yuskaitis at the Lookout Family Health Center in Morrison, Colorado, has been researching the tank for several years. His results have appeared in national medical journals. As reported in *Behavioral Medicine* magazine:

> Dr. Yuskaitis found that this method provided patients with the quickest reinforcement of the relaxation response. Most people don't know and have never experienced a complete state of relaxation . . . I found that many floating patients would, in a very short period of time learn the correct responses that accompany relaxation without resorting to long hours of meditation.

Dr. Yuskaitis has also used flotation successfully to wean chronic pain sufferers off of pain medications.

As for biofeedback, it too can be supplemented with flotation. Dr. Greg Jacobs at St. Elizabeth Hospital in Appleton, Wisconsin, studied 65 patients using R.E.S.T. and biofeedback. His results showed that the combination of the two produced a reduction of symptoms and improved patient's mood states. Ninety-one percent of the patients studied rated their condition as improved; 80 percent of the patients rated R.E.S.T. (floating) as more effective while only 20 percent rated biofeedback more effective.

Of course, once you are free of gravity, deep breathing can be done very effectively too, especially in overweight individuals who rarely experience good excursion of the diaphragm. A respiratory rate of only 3-4 breaths/min. is a frequent occurrence once someone has reached deep relaxation. Deep breathing will also hasten the meditative (alpha or theta) brainwave state.

Music is sometimes added: specific tapes designed for blood pressure reduction, muscle relaxation, etc. can be played on the underwater sound system available on most tanks. My most enjoyable experience occurred during the final three minutes of a float when I'd requested that the theme from *Chariots of Fire* be played over the speakers. The peripheral nerve endings on my skin had reset themselves to a lower threshhold of stimulation, which occurs to all receptors throughout the body in restricted sensory environments and explains why we experience our world to a greater degree after floating. Therefore, as the drums and trumpets began increasing in volume, I felt a tingling vibration all over my skin and experienced tremendous surges of energy flowing back and forth from head to toe. It was like a wild roller coaster ride compressed into ten seconds. After leaving the tank I felt refreshed and relaxed. I've never tried heroin or cocaine, but it's difficult to imagine surpassing that experience.

Finally, the visualization technique described in chapter 8 is greatly facilitated while in a R.E.S.T. condition, for two reasons. First, in the absence of other distractions it becomes easier to focus all our psychic energies and attention on visual material—video tapes, for example. By isolating the imagination alone to visualize goals, the body's other sensory channels are laid dormant and, especially when alpha is achieved, a more receptive state of mind is created in which total concentration occurs.

Second, "muscle memory programming" can occur. Simply stated, when the person views a perfectly executed skill, the brain imprints the electrical nerve-to-muscle sequence in its own memory file. When actual practice (or competition) takes place, the correct pattern of movement is executed almost automatically. Learning of motor skills thus can be accelerated by repeated viewing while in an otherwise relaxed, tension-free state. Does it really work? Three pro football teams think so and the testimonials continue to pile up from the likes of place kicker Raphael Septien, tennis player Stan Smith, and others.

Floating into the Future

So, where does all this leave us? It does *not* mean you cannot live without the use of a float tank, it does *not* mean you cannot learn to relax without one. This implication would be misleading. What it means is that you should do *something*! Experiment, try out the different approaches. Unless you resolve tension and/or other symptoms of distress you will be taking one huge risk, since peak performance and high-level wellness will continue to elude you. Things are not going to get any slower; they'll speed up as computer technology speeds up the flow of information. Therefore, I predict that the float tank will become an important wellness tool in the future as more research substantiates its need. By 1995, there will be a tank in every major medical center that promotes wellness. One in every 25 Americans will own one, since people will want the convenience of having one in their home. Who knows, maybe executive retreats will be held in elaborate float centers and an exotic date will involve partner shared floats with sumptuous wellness dinners post-floatem to tease those stimulation-hungry senses.

My own preference for the tank lies not only in its ability to produce immediate relaxation but because, as an antidote to boredom, it opens up a whole new frontier for exploring one's mind.

In the well acclaimed movie *Altered States*, a scientist enters a R.E.S.T. tank while on a hallucinogenic drug and emerges a flesh-eating savage. When asked to comment on this, Gary Higgins, President of Float To Relax (Lakewood, Colorado), responded, "We've never had a human go in the tank and come out as an animal, but we've had a lot of animals go in the tank and come out as humans."

Ever feel like the guy on the front cover of this book? Well, Gary's statement says it all.

Chapter 8
Selected References

Hutchinson, Michael. *The Book of Floating*. William Morrow & Co., 1984.

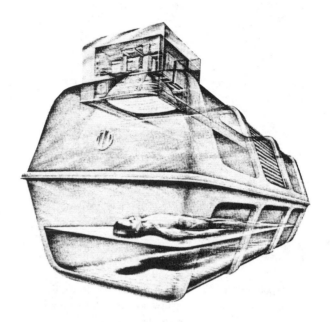

Restricted Environmental Stimulation Tanks (R.E.S.T.) can facilitate learning and promote deep states of relaxation.

Sensation Seeking: The Motivation To Risk

Self-exploration involves intelligent decision making. It means taking calculated risks, pursuing high-level wellness. We are all risk takers, but some of us are better at this game of life than others. Once you better understand some of the history and psychology of risk taking, you'll be more skilled at the wellness game, better able to control your own destiny. You won't make as many mistakes. You will be throwing loaded dice.

In the next chapter I will take you back in time very briefly to give you a feeling for life in antiquity when risk taking was a daily lesson in survival. Then, I will describe the differences between positive and negative risk taking so you can better evaluate the potential outcomes of your actions, relationships, and other uncertain events. Remember, as emphasized in the last section, *dis*-stress results from poor risk taking.

After you gain more insight into what risk taking is all about, you can break away from mediocrity and go exploring. The heroic goal will help you do this. The "flow experience" as an antidote to boredom should enlighten as well as open the door to many new life possibilities. Then, an analysis of why so many people fail to achieve happiness will follow. I'll relate this to some modern diseases and explore the fate of our nation.

CHAPTER 9
Historical Perspectives On Risk Taking

That which does not destroy you makes you strong.
—Friedrich Nietzsche

Imagine yourself for a moment, thrust backward in time, some 80,000 years ago. Deep within a limestone cave you awaken to a still crackling fire, intensely hungry like the other members of your tribe, for you have not eaten for almost three days. The bones strewn about you have been picked clean and even the snakeheads have been long eaten. Beset by another tribe of hunters who tried to kill your tribe for the fire—a source of power since it gave control over nature—your tribal family has stayed within the confines of the cave, unwilling to venture out. But hunger now has created another kind of fear. Getting to your feet and taking your flint ax in one hand and your spear in another, you waken two tribesmen. They willingly arise, grab their weapons and silently follow, for they too know the feelings of an empty gut. One tribesman throws some dried dog dung upon the fire to keep it going.

Together, you risk going outside. Crouching low so as to make for a smaller target for a flying spear, you venture out into the small open space between the cave and surrounding brush. First you retrieve your dead, five tribesmen slain during the fighting several days earlier. Then carefully you move toward the brush, eyes watching for the slightest movement. Periodically you pause to tilt your head upward, smell of unfamiliar others (your smell at that time was very keen). You listen intently for a few moments. You walk farther until you reach a rock-laden hillside. Looking down, all seems well, your enemy seems to have departed. Another risk now seems imminent, for now you must stalk and kill an animal large enough to feed the tribe, but your energy reserves are low, and your enemy might return.

This scene, similar to one portrayed in the popular movie, *Quest For*

Fire, depicts the harshness of living in that age. As in the movie, the threat to survival was an omnipotent fact of life for early humans for they had to battle the weather, the terrain, and other living creatures to stay alive. Most of their waking hours were spent in search of food, water, and shelter. Avoiding or fighting their enemies was an ever-present reality. For our primitive ancestors, it was not a question of whether or not to take risks; they had to in order to survive.

Defining Risk Taking

It is critical to redefine this term, *risk taking,* before embarking on a historical perspective of the concept. The word "risk" has assumed rather negative connotations. It is true that the term is best defined as a situation where loss or gain may occur. The gambling of what you have for something more, to chance losing all is another way of phrasing it. Risking something is the *sine qua non* for a win to occur, and the satisfaction it brings. It's the more negative or loss possibilities that tend to color the use of the word "risk."

To risk, to take chances, has long been equated with impulsiveness, recklessness, and even insanity. Daredevils or chronic thrill-seekers were generally seen as having some type of death wish. This narrow, and perhaps inaccurate, conception of risk taking, however, has been undergoing rapid changes in the last ten to fifteen years. It's proving to be a psychological concept long overdue for recognition as central to human behavior.

The "gain" side of the ledger can lead to a much healthier and happier lifestyle, so much so that it is truly amazing that risk taking as a form of human behavior has been unexamined and unappreciated for so lng.

Risk taking in its many forms is as old as human history. Many primitive religions were built around the taking of risks, of enduring deprivation as rites of passage into adulthood. Male Hopi youths would journey through the canyon of the Little Colorado River and across a wide expanse of the Arizona desert before attempting a treacherous climb to a salt cave high on the canyon wall.

Tibetan lamas and Nepalese shamans have long participated in ritualistic mountain climbing at the highest elevations on earth. Manchu medicine men of Northeastern China would chop several widely spaced holes in a frozen river and then dive under the ice and swim to see if they could find the scattered exits they had made in the ice. Jamaican holy men would swim as far out to sea as possible, then turn and try to make it back. Melanesian men dive from 70-foot towers with vines tied to their feet just long enough to break their fall inches from the ground. Such rituals or feats were often performed to induce a meditative state through fasting, ordeal, and exhaustion. Our modern day triathlons demonstrate that such traditions and needs in people are not dead.

In every culture, whether sanctioned or not, there have been individuals who pushed to the limits and beyond. With the advent of the Age of Reason, and the Industrial Revolution, where rational thinking and the experimental method were highly valued, the person who behaved without regard to costs and risks was considered irrational. The advancement of human civilization may in part be described as an endeavor to displace the nonrational with rational actions. Over the centuries, an ever-changing blend of the rational aspects of human nature has coexisted with the nonrational.

Most religions, with their powerful forces and economic ties, have supported the rational approach to human behavior. Wild, impulsive behavior was seen as disobedience to the common order and surely the mark of evil influence.

Friedrich Nietzsche, the German philosopher, said that everything in human life has two poles, the Dionysian and the Apollonian. The Dionysian is God and nature's primal strength, the unending turbulent lust and longing in man that drives him to conquest, to dare, to love, to mystic ecstasy. The Apollonian, on the other hand, is an attempt to stop this unending struggle, to find peace, harmony, balance, and to restrain the wild, unpredictable impulses. Society and its laws and mores comes down forcefully on the side of the Apollonian.

The life force represented in the Dionysian side of human nature, however, is not easily subverted. The anticipation and excitement of entering the arena, of winning or losing, creeps into many areas of life. Business enterprises do not exist solely for the pursuit of profits. For many wealthy people, the satisfaction is in the drama and gamesmanship of the transaction. Organized sports and games are not simply played for the victory. The anticipation prior to the contest and intensity of the given activity often far outweighs who wins and who loses for spectators *and* participants alike. Crimes often have a thrill-seeking element and are not just a short-cut to economic gains. Even wars between countries occur for reasons other than capturing markets or protecting living space. The factor of engaging in an exciting, suspenseful, exhilarating endeavor colors most of human behavior, both in individuals and collective groups.

Pitting oneself against the unknown, the resistant forces of life, is quite common. Some seek the challenge of the natural environment. Exploring rugged, uncharted terrain or building an extended tunnel through a granite mountain reflect this type of challenge.

Creating an aesthetic entity out of an amorphous mass or a blank canvas is another form of stepping into the unknown and seeing what develops. Creativity, in its infinite forms of expression, always involves some form of risk taking, of seeing things in a different, original manner. It is certainly not the static forces of the status quo that breed creative behavior.

Learning itself involves having an open mind, a willingness to consider new information—thesis, antithesis, leading to a synthesis. Daring to experiment, to attempt something new, forms the basis of advancing civilization—not the staid, regimented Apollonian emphasis. Pioneers must have a frontier to challenge their minds and bodies.

Risk Taking as Necessary to Life

Why has the concept of risk taking been ignored in the social sciences when its effects are so pervasive? Psychology has long built its theories around a stress-reduction or homeostatic model of behavior. In other words, anything arousing or exciting must be reduced in order to maintain a balanced condition in the body. In 1915, Sigmund Freud wrote:

> The nervous system is an apparatus having the function of abolishing stimuli which reach it or of reducing excitation to the lowest possible level; an apparatus which would, if this were feasible, maintain itself in an altogether unstimulated condition.

This line of thinking, along with several other theories of reducing or avoiding stimulation, defined human behavior for the social sciences until 1954 when sensory deprivation research at McGill University in Canada drove a solid wedge into these established theories. In the late 1940s D. O. Hebb, a psychophysiologist, stated that stimulation of at least moderate intensity is needed to keep the human being satisfied and in touch with reality. It wasn't until the research at McGill University, which purposefully reduced stimulation to its lowest possible level (sensory deprivation), that Hebb's contentions were substantiated. Human subjects deprived of normal levels of sound, touch, and visual stimuli showed their displeasure by reacting very strongly to this condition. Some simply left the tests early; others exhibited classical psychotic behavior (hallucinations, body-image distortions, etc.). It appears that if external stimuli is not presented to the subjects, they will create their own! *Risk taking will be internalized.*

Two other historical events of the 1950s substantiated the sensory deprivation research. Our troops had just returned from Korea with horror stories about the effectiveness of Chinese brainwashing. Many of these mind-bending techniques involved long periods of isolation and deprivation followed by sessions of propaganda. Was it restricted confinement or the propaganda that had such a powerful effect? The former possibility made more sense in view of the MGill research.

The second major human enterprise of the Fifties that spurred interest in man's apparent need for stimulation was the Mercury Astronaut program. What were America's finest going to do up there in space cut off from everything familiar? The project could be seriously jeopardized if the astronauts exhibited the unusual reactions of the McGill research subjects.

Hebb's earlier conjecture about the need for stimulation took on new credibility in the light of this research from the lab and field. Humans must certainly have "preprogrammed" needs for stimulus-seeking and selecting novel information. New and varied life experiences appeared necessary to maintain the organization and functioning of the nervous system. Stimulation not only proved to create learned behavioral responses but to spark the essence of life itself. We need stimulation, and risk taking in its various forms serves this function.

Since this early research of the Fifties, risk taking as a legitimate topic of scientific research has found its place. Risk taking has been viewed from many perspectives in man and lower animals, though most of this has been confined to the artificial environment of laboratories. Some sample research titles are: "Polynomial Psychophysics of Group Risk Perception", "Socio-Psychological Dynamics of Risk Taking Behavior", and "Advisement to Take Risks—The Elderly's View". Though risk taking has been examined in many everyday behaviors, such as driving, smoking, etc., such research rarely focuses upon extreme forms of risk taking.

Let us return to the impact of social forces on risk taking behavior. On the one hand, as civilization has progressed, it has become more regimented and predictable, while on the other hand, our society provides us with an ever-increasing array of stimuli. The battle for the consumer dollar is very dependent on two factors: first, attracting the public's attention via some form of stimulus; then the product or service being sold must deliver, it must stimulate in some novel, and often intense, manner.

The result of this "sensational" battle for the consumers' dollars is the creation of a human being that expects—even needs—ever-increasing levels of stimulation. One psychologist stated that an alarming number of people in this country may be tabbed "excitement addicts." These people crave daily crises and risky events just as a heroin addict needs a fix. Job dissatisfaction is often a major cause of this craving for excitement to counter the repetitive, boring routine. Feeling locked into a monotonous existence, these people yearn to break out and try something new— something stimulating, challenging, and personally rewarding.

Television may be a major culprit in this exponential need to attempt daring and novel experiences. Instant entertainment on television tends to condition people to be passive spectators. As the research indicates, this runs counter to the normal human condition. Thus, people can only be expected to feel the urge to break out of this passive, dronelike state of mind to a more active involvement in life.

Video games provide for more participation and challenge. With the new home screen videos, the fear of addiction and mind warping are issued. Many youths pursue the arcade and home style computer games with an obsession, thus confirming the fears of many. For generations raised on a steady diet of television, the video games do apparently satisfy the need to participate and control the action on the screen. Other common outlets for this need for intense excitement are the multibillion dollar industry of gambling and the even more common activity of buying behavior. Buying something new is a tried-and-true way of reducing boredom, at least temporarily, by bringing something new into one's life. When all else fails, mind-altering drugs or involvement in some cultist movement may produce the desired stimulation.

Primitive people existed at or near their optimal arousal level on a daily basis. Their needs were simple and concrete, and they were kept busy meeting them. Modern men and women, on the other hand, in their protected and predictable environment, often find themselves either over- or understimulated. Thus, they alternate between attending stress management seminars and asking travel agents about new, exciting places to visit.

It's true we're free to choose our activities, whereas our primitive counterparts were bound by survival needs. But the task of experiencing just enough stimulation is a complex one. Many people simply give up and lead lives of mundane routine. No hits, no runs, no errors.

The Question of Self-exploration

The cost of giving up on personal growth and taking that daring step into the unknown is a high one. We can shut ourselves off in some type of artificial cocoon and wait for death, or we can venture out. Too much of the former can lead to a deadening type of isolation and non-feeling. Rod Steiger, in his dramatic portrayal in *The Pawnbroker,* in a desperate attempt to feel something in his shallow, cut-off existence, finally forces his hand slowly through a paper-spindle just to feel something. Lives of quiet desperation can be had by many people in our modern, urban society. The common malady of depression gains much strength from inactivity and predictable, meaningless outcomes.

Breaking out of a passive, boring, redundant lifestyle can do wonders for one's mind and body. That which gives you safety, security, familiarity, the necessary ingredients which, in moderation, keep you sane, should be abandoned when they start to contract and harden into the static, the confining, and the outgrown. The poison of self-paralysis acts slowly but, like that of a brown recluse spider, is just as certain.

What to let go of? It can be a less-than-satisfying job, a bankrupt marriage, your eating and drinking habits, even your self-image. Many things, often comfortable companions, can keep us restricted and erode our wellness.

The life force is powerful and relentless, thrusting us forward and challenging the need for safety. The need for security, however, is also quite strong and can provide stiff resistance to our desire for freedom from the status quo. The known, however unsatisfying, is certain, quite unlike the threat of the unknown.

It is for each to decide the costs of risking, in hopes of greater gain, or accepting life as adequate. Throughout history, however, it has become clear that, by taking risks, a new, more vivid world can be experienced, something so real that you may return again and again for the sensation.

CHAPTER 9
Selected References

Lowe, Robert A. *Primitive Religions*. Liveright Publications, 1970.

CHAPTER 10

Risk Taking: Art or Science?

I love to take risks—not risks that aren't calculated, but risks that I sit down and calculate. What do I have to gain, what is the actual risk, what's the worst that can happen, and can I live with it.

—Brooke Knapp, female holder of 105 world-class speed records in aviation, including circumnavigation of the globe.

Being a good risk taker in today's world isn't easy. We're hit with a barrage of ads in one form or another, all with the implied message, "Without _____you are less, this will make you a better, happier, more together person."

Decisions regarding risk are astronomical. Do we drink diet soda containing cyclamates? Are tampons really safe? Will the Pill cause any long-term side effects? Should I fly or drive the 150 miles? Should I risk driving home after drinking all evening? Can I continue smoking as I have for 15 years without worrying about a heart attack? Should I tell _____my feelings and let her know how much I really care? Should I gamble all my savings on this business venture or leave my money in the bank? When you stop and think about it, almost everything we do from the time we get out of bed until we shut our eyes that evening involves decisions about risk taking in some form or another.

The question is, can risks be managed; can they be predicted and controlled for; can we take control of our own destiny? I believe we can. This is really what wellness is all about, taking responsibility for your actions. I don't believe there's a God who sits on high and punches a central keyboard saying whose time it is to go, and where, and when. I believe God gave us the great gift of insight, of the ability to use our intellect to analyze the risks we take every day. I survived my high-risk activities because I was meticulous and systematic in managing the various risks so that the odds were much in my favor. But I also know that human beings are *not* strictly rational creatures and often act on their emotions at a particular time. For example, 50 percent of Americans are overweight. Being overweight is statistically related to almost all of our noncommunicable diseases, like heart disease, cancer, diabetes, and strokes. And yet, how many of us, upon entering the cafeteria line and passing the custard creme pie, cheesecake, or German chocolate cake will abstain because we know it adds to our risk?

I believe risk taking is a vital part of life. If your goal is high-level wellness, then you'll have to take some big risks, since this will mean leaving present comfort zones behind, giving up bad habits, developing new behaviors that allow you to reach greater heights, physically *and* spiritually. There are always obstacles, but a positive risk taker learns how to get over them.

Think about some of the risks I took to reach my goal of testing my limits, and gathering the material for this book. I risked lost income. I risked being thought crazy. Of course I care what people think, but my own happiness was more important than trying to live up to society's norms and expectations. Besides, I was having fun. Experienced-based learning taught me a lot about the relationship of risk taking to wellness. I have used much of this knowledge to motivate some of the corporate clientele I work with as a wellness consultant.

The following table will help you understand how behaviors determine low-or high-level wellness. Examples are provided.

Risk Taking Behaviors Can Determine Your Wellness

Risk Behaviors	LOW-LEVEL WELLNESS *Negative Risk Taking*	OR	HIGH-LEVEL WELLNESS *Positive Risk Taking*
Physical	Reckless driving, alcohol abuse, smoking, overeating, drug abuse, nonuse of seat belts, high sugar and caffeine intake. Lack of exercise		Walking/jogging, skiing, canoeing, roller skating, mountain climbing, or any kind of sport for promoting endurance and enhancing strength.
Social	Poor communication of thoughts, crime, and violent aggression. Extreme introversion, destructive criticism. Expending great energy creating status symbols		Good listening skills. Meeting new people, (you risk conversation), being assertive, constructive criticism. Laughing, crying, comfortable clothes worn out of fashion.
Emotional	Anger held in or any form of bottled up emotions. Extra-marital sex.		Some kinds of music. Expressing your inner feelings verbally or by touch (hugging). Saying, "I love you."

Risk Behaviors	LOW-LEVEL WELLNESS OR	HIGH-LEVEL WELLNESS
	Negative Risk Taking	*Positive Risk Taking*
Mental	Pornographic films or literature, too much TV, habitual gambling, video games?, poorly conceived business ventures, always in a race with the clock, Negative attitudes	Educational pursuits, travel, any creative challenge like art, writing, inventing, well-conceived business ventures. Any stress control technique like meditation Prayer

First let me explain the difference between positive and negative risk taking. Then I'll describe each main type of risk.

Negative risks are self-defeating because definite and predictable health hazards are involved. They move you in the direction of illness and usually provide only immediate gratification. *Positive* risks move you in the wellness direction. They promote increased physical fitness, increased self-confidence, better friendships (social supports), and help you achieve high goals in both business and personal areas.

Positive risks provide a healthy psychological outlet to satisfy our innate need for stimulation and relief from boredom. They're growth opportunities because they foster a well-rounded, happier, and fulfilled person. The satisfactions and heightened arousal levels they provide last much longer.

Physical Risk Taking

When I first began doing the feats in the spring of 1979, I contacted the Stuntmen's Association of Motion Pictures in Hollywood. I thought I'd better talk to the people who do this kind of thing as a profession. I recall talking to a stuntman named Conrad Palmisano. I asked him, "How do you know when you are ready, I mean when the stunt is ready to go?"

He answered, "Gut reaction. You just get a gut feeling about whether or not it's going to work. If you don't feel right about it, then something somewhere isn't right and you keep working on it."

Now, although I could appreciate what he was saying, having studied the scientific method in my research courses, I know there is always a scientific way of looking at a problem, especially when that problem is going to keep recurring. In research methodology this is called *analysis of variance*, a fancy way of saying, "Let's see if we can find certain key factors that will help predict the occurrence of an event." For example, if we performed an analysis of variance on car accidents, looking at a

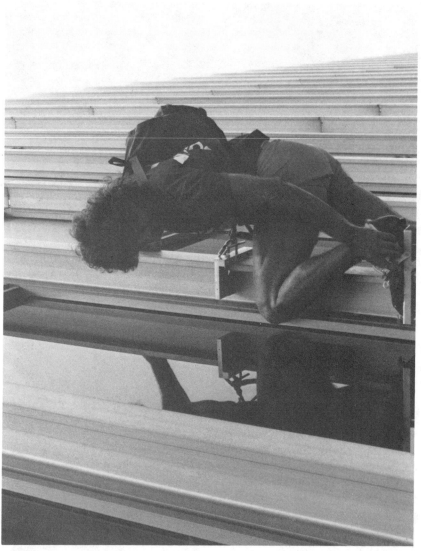

Risk taking is both an art and a science. You analyze the risks, you develop a plan, you establish "back-up" systems, you stay fit, and the chances are great you will succeed.

variety of factors or situations that were highly associated with car accidents, we might uncover some interesting pieces of information. We might discover that most car accidents occur during rush-hour traffic or on holidays. We might also discover that many accidents happen to single people under 25 years of age. Then, if we wanted to predict the risk of a car accident, we could combine all three of these findings and state that for any given year, approximately 70 percent of all traffic accidents will occur in bad weather, during periods of heavy traffic flow, to those under 25 years of age. If this guesstimate (*hypothesis,* we call it) turns out to be fairly accurate, we have then gained some measure of control over the risk of a car accident. This is because now we can state some of the conditions that increase the likelihood of an accident. This kind of control is very valuable because we can then save lives by cautioning people to be extra careful at those times. In primitive times, the risks were clearly defined and fairly obvious. But in a highly complex society, most risks are hidden. In a recent Louis Harris survey (*"Risk in a Complex Society"*) this fact was brought out, along with data that show that most people want to be informed. They want to know what the risks are so they have a measure of control over life, so they can deal with Technological Shock Syndrome. Forty thousand years ago, if one of our ancestors bent over to drink from a stream, he didn't have to worry whether or not someone upstream had dumped some chemical in the water. Incidently, a recent EPA study on over 850 cities in the United States found that in 29 percent of those cities the water was unfit for human consumption. This brings us to rule number one in becoming a good risk taker.

Rule 1. Investigate as much as possible all the factors related to your safety. In research these are called risk factors.

For any area of risk taking, this information is almost always available in periodicals and other publications: (*American Health, Harvard Medical Newsletter, Executive Health,* etc.) You just need to go about finding it. For example, prior to my years as a graduate student, I was pretty much like most of my readers. I didn't think a lot about risk taking. I usually based decisions on how I felt at the time. Once I began studying disease prevention, I learned that for every major disease there exist risk factors, events or actions (behaviors) that increase the odds of developing a disease. For example, if a person smokes at least one pack of cigarettes per day their risk of heart disease goes up five times the normal rate. If they also show a very high level of fat or sugar in their blood the risk becomes 20 times normal. This information has been gathered from extensive research conducted over the last 25 years.

What I'm saying is this: Let's suppose the example just given was your spouse or one of your parents. The odds finally caught up with them and they died at a fairly young age, say 58. Everyone would gather at the home of the dearly departed, grieve for awhile, cry at the funeral, and then conclude that "God must have figured it was time for him to leave."

Hogwash! Neither God, nor Jesus, nor any of the Holy Scriptures ever said a person should smoke or should eat food loaded with fat, sugar, or salt. Don't blame God for man's indignities and insults to a body He designed to last a hundred years. To do so is a cop-out of the worst kind. This is why I've listed such things as smoking, alcohol abuse, and nonuse of seatbelts under negative risk taking.

As a former life insurance examiner, I'm convinced most of us live under the illusion that we control risks when, in fact, the risk is controlling us. An example should prove my point.

It's often happened in the course of my risky adventures that someone will come up to me and say something like, "Man, you really have a lot of guts. I could *never* do anything that risky." I then begin a series of questions which, by the time I am finished, demonstrates to that person the fact that he is taking a lot of risks which, for the most part, he was unaware of. As dramatic and dangerous as my extreme sports have appeared, I've still been in control of the risks. Why? Because I analyzed each one very carefully in terms of the risk factors, trying to foresee possible problems. I'd then gradually try to eliminate the problems, either by correcting for equipment and experience or manipulating the environment in some way. All I've done in this book is apply the risk-factor concept to all aspects of life, since wellness means controlling those things which relate to optimal health. There's an important lesson here regarding risk taking. It becomes rule number two.

Rule 2   We tend to think of something as risky or dangerous only if the risk is readily apparent. This is simply *not* true. *Many risks are hidden!*

One more example. Almost everyone thinks skydiving is dangerous. Why? Because the risk is so frighteningly obvious. You are opening up the door of an airplane several thousand feet above Earth. There is no denying the possible outcome. In fact, the intensity of the situation is so scary you'd do everything you possibly could to make sure you are fully prepared for the jump. On the other hand, you don't perceive that one cigarette will kill you. *One* certainly won't. It's not very intense, picking up a three-ounce white cylinder of paper-filled with tobacco and inhaling deep into your lungs. But you cannot see into your lungs, arteries, and heart so you think you are in control; you can quit before the odds catch up to you. So consider this next little tidbit of information if you've been doing it at least 10–20 years. According to Kansas City Life Insurance actuaries, they'll charge a 50-year-old skydiving non-smoking male $3.00 per $1,000 of life insurance he applies for. But, if he is a 50-year-old non-skydiving smoker, they will charge him $9.00 per $1,000 of life insurance. So who is the daredevil? According to data I was able to gather, there is about one skydiving death per every 42,000 jumps. These are better odds than smoking. But, you may be sure that every one of those deaths will make the newspaper. It is dramatic, like my high-risk activities were. Some drinking drivers might make the newspapers. This is also more intense. And what about our racing executive, who has high blood pressure, smokes, and has high cholesterol? Is his risk greater than the USAC formula race car driver? Yes, by a factor of almost ten. According to information provided by USAC, the risk of death in ten years is about 3/100. According to American Heart Association data, the 45-year-old racing executive has a 3/10 chance of dying in the next ten years. But, the formula race-car driver is the daredevil. Truth is, he *manages* the risks. The executive doesn't.

How do you discern the physical risk factors? Fortunately, all this work has been done for you. Most of the risk factors for many major diseases and accidents are included in the Life Risk Questionnaire in chapter 1.

These risk factors are under your control since they're heavily influenced by the lifestyle you choose. The choices you make determine the odds. As a former life insurance examiner, I assure you this questionnaire is far more comprehensive and predictive of your future health than the typical questionnaires I administered to insurance clients. Many of the risk factors are also included in a questionnaire at the conclusion of this chapter so you may estimate your life expectancy.

For those who simply want to know the state-of-the-art, risk factors for two of our more common diseases are listed here.

Risk Factors For Cancer, risk factors include:
- High fat diets
- Low fiber diets (less than 37 grams)
- Low vitamin A diets
- Low vitamin C diets (evidence very suggestive)
- Caffeine?
- Smoking
- *Dis*-stress (depression, despair)
- Known carcinogenic agents (nitrates, coal, tar, and many many others)
- Excessive intake of refined sugars
- The contraceptive pill

Some Risk Factors for Heart Disease are:
- Smoking
- Obesity
- High blood pressure
- High blood fats (cholesterol and triglycerides)
- High blood sugar
- Family history of circulatory problems
- Lack of exercise
- *Dis*-stress (Type-A behavior pattern)
- Oral contraceptives
- Caffeine (evidence very suggestive)

As for the so-called risky sports, such as white-water canoeing, or hang gliding, there also exist risk factors that should be considered in order to make them enjoyable, positive, character-building experiences. In the past three years I've tried white-water canoeing, rock climbing, ultralight flying, scuba diving, cliff jumping, skydiving, cross-country skiing, and mountain motocross. For most of these sports I gathered a lot of information on fatalities in order to tease out the risk factors, since some of these involved my own survival. What did I find? Each sport has a set of safety guidelines, although many times the death victim ignored them. When you decide to get into such sports, take the necessary training, find out all you can about safety and possible hazards, and progress slowly so skill development is parallel with the increasing challenges.

From my experience in a variety of high-risk activities, I have found out that many deaths occur because the participant did not have a back-up system—an alternate plan of action should something fail. It has wide application to many areas of life. It becomes rule number three.

Rule 3. Whenever you are preparing to take a major risk, where potential losses may be great, leave yourself an out, *have a back-up plan* should your primary plan fail.

This rule applies regardless of whether the risk is physical, social, emotional, or financial. Remember when I described my 9000-foot first-time freefall? Recall that the parachute failed to open. I not only had another skydiver in the air with me (who had over 3,000 jumps and was a four-time world champion) but I had the best possible equipment, which included an automatic 22-activated opener for the reserve parachute just in case I had frozen from fear. This automatic opener isn't perfect (80 percent reliability) but did represent another of the back-up systems available to me.

So I read about two white-water canoeists who drowned last Memorial Day. I look for risk factors. What do I find? They weren't wearing life vests, they'd been drinking heavily, and they were inexperienced canoeists in rapidly moving water. So three risk factors were present: they were unprepared and they had no back-up system in the form of life vests. Is it any wonder they died? Is this an act of God or of man?

Social-Emotional Risk Taking

Whenever I am speaking to groups of people on the subject of positive risk taking, I always try to convey the notion that risk taking is a very broad category that also includes going outside your normal social setting to meet new people. We don't usually tend to think of this as risk taking in the same sense as physical risk taking. Still, many of the same principles apply. We're taking a chance, with something to gain (payoff) and something to lose. The payoff can be the enrichment of sharing new experiences, learning new things, and growing more through the other person. When I surveyed employees at a life insurance company, I found that much of the distress involved not having enough close friends, not being able to say what they feel to either their spouse or supervisor, and performing unwanted tasks because they didn't know how to say no. To overcome these difficulties and obstacles, to pull your own strings, requires that you become a good social-emotional risk taker. Yes, if you open up to someone you can get hurt, you expose your real feelings and you're more vulnerable. But what good is life if you never give yourself an opportunity to grow, to share, to love deeply? You're only half alive, cut off from letting the real you be discovered.

Now, let's see how some of the same principles apply. Remember we will begin by looking for risk factors, those things that can represent potential problems. If you wish to expand your friendships and enhance your emotional relationships with significant others, you can begin preparing for the risk by first doing some self-examination. Self-examination is always the first step to achieving high-level wellness. Ask yourself questions: Who am I? What am I? Where am I going? What are my goals? What things are important to me in life? Once you can answer these questions, you will have a better perspective on yourself. Then, you will be able to reduce the social-emotional risk factors and risk moving toward those people, or groups of people, who share your same interests, preferences, and goals. In other words, the odds of developing friendships and deep emotional attachments won't be good if the individuals you attract are going in different directions. An example should help.

Susan worked an eight-hour day as a secretary for a large construction company. Only two other women worked for this company; both were married and had families. Susan didn't drink and didn't make a really big salary, so she wasn't into the bar scene after work. She usually went home and spent the evening watching TV or occasionally reading a book. Sometimes she went to see her family and sometimes she went shopping. For the most part, she described her life as very boring and very lonely. She asked herself the question posed earlier and came to the realization that she wanted to lose weight and also wanted to pursue her interest in art and photography. She joined a spa where she went three or four evenings per week and enrolled in an art course at night school. Her life took on new meaning. She was finally happy to be physically active and her art provided a creative challenge she needed.

Susan also came in contact with a lot of new people at both places by "risking" conversation and suggesting they do something together. She even met a young man who shared her interest in art and photography and they spent a lot of time doing nature trips. She has opened up to him about her feelings and she is sure to let him know her true feelings on certain issues regarding sex, music, and art, even if it differs from his.

Thus, Susan will now be able to expand herself a lot more, and grow emotionally and socially from her new friendships. She took some risks but she took well-calculated ones. Her friendships arose out of a consideration of her own goals and her own sense of direction. In this way she was decreasing the chance of rejection, of not being accepted. She asserted herself and communicated openly so her new friends would know where she stood. Also, she had a back-up system: she maintained her friendships outside of her boyfriend, and kept close family ties. By opening up her emotions she took a risk by expressing her views. But this was a positive risk because her emotions would not get bottled up to a boiling point—a negative risk.

One of the most difficult things is to assert oneself, to communicate one's deepest feelings. "I might get hurt." Surely you may. But you'll never know unless you risk. I've been hurt deeply. But I've known the joys of love also. Such experiences, good and bad, have made me a deeper, more loving, more sensitive person. What would life be with no hits, no runs, no errors? High-level wellness means giving up mediocrity.

Other possible risk factors to consider in this area might be things like stability, consistency, and honesty. Are you doing all the opening up? Or is your partner also opening up their feelings? Perhaps the biggest risk factor of all in this category would be expectancies. What do you expect? What does your partner expect? It's wise to uncover this as soon as possible in a relationship. Your partner may not be ready for anything serious. You may be. So, if you risk revealing everything you feel, you may be taking a pretty big risk. It's great to feel deeply and let your partner know, but if he/she doesn't share the same expectancy in terms of marriage, a one-to-one dating relationship, etc., the outcome could hurt quite a bit. Define the relationships. Remember your back-up systems. Have an alternative plan. Don't put all your eggs in one basket unless you are very sure the basket can hold them all! Maintain family-friend relationships.

Some of the social-emotional risk factors are:
- Different goals
- Different expectancies
- Unstable personality
- Inconsistency
- Dishonesty
- Different value systems
- Low self-esteem
- Job dissatisfaction
- Unstable family life or parents

Look at the track record of the friends and close acquaintances you are making. Are they dependable? Can you rely on them? Do they just want to conquer someone who represents a challenge? What are their life priorities, their value systems? How often we've heard someone say, "I found out I didn't really know her at all." I'll ask, "How hard did you look or did you see what you wanted to see?" One of the most difficult of all things to predict is how a human being will react. We can easily predict physical phenomena, but human behavior is one of the most difficult things to understand fully. Still, we must risk. Dr. David Viscott, in his excellent book, *Risking,* tells why we must risk closeness even if the possible outcome is pain.

> In a risk of love you must risk for yourself. Any risk you take must improve your chances of becoming you. A risk of love that restricts the ability to grow into your best self is no risk at all, but a self-destructive act that does not increase your freedom. . . . To risk for the love of another person without risking for the love of yourself is to set up a failure in the future when your needs surface and demand to be fulfilled. . . . If you don't protect your rights in taking a risk of love, you'll undermine the very love you risk for.

Dr. Viscott then provides some good guidelines for a successful risk of love.

1. A risk of love succeeds when it allows a person to grow.
2. A risk of love succeeds when it allows two people to share the most special parts of themselves.
3. A risk of love succeeds when it allows a person to accept his faults and to value himself in spite of them.
4. A risk of love succeeds when a person can risk everything and lose, but still believes they came out ahead because they became more open and now knows more about themselves.

The last of these guidelines requires a great deal of courage. The last three years of my life have been a period of great emotional turmoil, but I regard as my most courageous act, not the ability to jump from a high bridge span or from an airplane but once again to risk the words, "I love you very much," and "You're special to me, I care about you."

Dr. Maslow, the psychologist who pioneered high-level wellness by studying the "supernormal personality," stated that self-actualized people have a good grasp upon their self-identity, they don't feel they're giving anything away by "letting their hair down, by telling their partner their deepest fears and weaknesses," but rather that the idea of self-delusion and self-deception are simply not part of their behavioral repertoire. They need no facade, they feel familiarity does not breed contempt, but rather an excursion into the inner beauty, since they are receptive to all of life's experiences, good and bad.

> My people report that they can be themselves without feeling that there are demands or expectations placed upon them; they can feel psychologically (as well as physically) naked and still feel loved and wanted and secure.

Mental and Financial Risk Taking

I've given examples of educational pursuits, travel, etc. The longer you stay in school the more you're risking in terms of finances and time. However, almost nothing else has the guaranteed payoffs of advanced education, although this is considerably less true today than in the past. People seeking high-level wellness recognize that intellectual growth is just as important to self-development as is physical growth. Our value systems are to a large degree dependent upon the kind of thoughts we put into our minds.

Even in choosing a career, we need to investigate for risk factors. Some jobs are in high demand, for example, in computer technology and electrical engineering. The U.S. Department of Labor publication, *Occupational Outlook Handbook,* describes over 1,000 jobs, listing average salaries and job descriptions. It would be a mistake, however, to select a job or career strictly on the basis of its earnings. Personal satisfaction and growth opportunities are other considerations.

Vocational counselors can perform extensive tests to help you identify your aptitude in a wide range of areas. Temper information with existing realities when making your final decision. For example, says Thomas C. Devlin, Director of Cornell University's Career Center, "The American Dream of getting a degree in one hand and a job in the other has been deteriorating."

Jack Shingleton, Placement Director at Michigan State University, states, "Universities are turning out more graduates than our society is able to absorb."

The federal government's Scientific Manpower Commission predicts that in 1992 there will be 3.3 million more graduates than jobs requiring a college degree. The 1983 graduates most in demand by corporations were those in electrical engineering, computer science, and accounting. Conditions change, however, and the once-booming market for engineers is down 18 percent from 1982. Stay tuned to trends.

According to the College Placement Council, liberal arts students face the bleakest prospects of all, with average starting salaries down 7 percent from 1982 levels to $14,256. Counselors are predicting that liberal arts students without highly specialized skills will have a frustrating time finding jobs and may end up accepting low-pay, low-prestige jobs. To offset this, many colleges require them to take additional courses such as accounting and computer science to give them more versatility and diversity.

Grades are always a consideration, and many companies place great emphasis upon grade-point averages as a criterion for hiring. However, experience and diversity may be more important to many companies. I'd highly recommend gaining any experience you can during summers, and other breaks even if it means giving up some income. This effort communicates desire and ambition to prospective employers.

Remember, if you select a job purely on the basis of money, you've sealed your fate, one likely to be marked with boredom, discontent, and unfulfillment. Where there's no satisfaction, you will have little or no enthusiasm. One study found that the amount of job stress perceived was not related to the pace of the job but rather the degree of monotony present. Bored employees had twice the heart attack rate as those performing jobs that offered lots of task variety. Keep that in mind. So, now let me summarize the educational and career placement risk factors to consider when you are trying to enter the job market.

- Attitude (generate enthusiasm)
- Personal appearance (fat versus fit)
- Quality of college attended
- Grade-point average
- Specific field chosen (some more in demand)
- Communication skills
- Diversity of academic background
- Experience in chosen field
- Number of contacts made (perseverance factor)
- Interview and resume skills
- Personal satisfaction with chosen field

As emphasized before, the last of these may be the most important consideration of all.

Because I frequently lecture to various business groups, I try to bridge the gap between my feats and success in business by telling them many of the same risk-taking concepts apply. For example, at a talk to two hundred restaurant owners, I asked questions like, "What would you do if you were catering a large function and one of your ovens broke down? What would you do if half of your help didn't show up because of the flu? What if a large shipment of beef failed to arrive?"

Many had alternate back-up systems, as in rule three. They knew where else they could get supplies on short notice and/or they had other people they could call on to fill in for regular employees. Some, however, hadn't really given any thought to a crisis situation. They hadn't anticipated rule one, recognize your risk factors or potential problems. Remember Murphy's first law: "If anything can go wrong, it most certainly will."

I asked them how important location was. I asked them if they knew there was a computer service which for $300.00 would conduct a market research survey on where a restaurant could locate to have its best chance. This service had a success record of 95 percent. It would look at the type of food being served, style of food service (cafeteria, etc.), income level of the area, amount of traffic flow, and many other risk factors, in order to predict how well the restaurant would fare in the next five years. I told them their health would affect their success because they'd handle job stresses better in the same way I handled my stresses better.

Any financial risk requires thorough investigation and market surveys in the same way I thoroughly investigated my risks in order to succeed. But remember Rule Two: many risks are hidden. This is apt to be especially true when the venture is of a new type. John DeLorean attempted to do what no one in the automobile industry had done since Henry J. Kaiser in the 1940s: start an auto company and compete successfully in a market dominated by Ford, Chrysler, and General Motors. Although DeLorean's market research was not very promising, he avidly pursued his dream. His daring venture didn't seem to succeed, although experts admit it might have succeeded ten years earlier. This brings us to the fourth and last rule of risk taking:

Rule 4. Timing is all important. Something may work or succeed at one time and yet fail at another time.

This rule tends to hold true in personal relationships or business ventures. Change is constant. Nothing stays the same. Try to maintain a sense of time consciousness in your risk taking. Don't become too secure; stay in touch with trends but don't be ruled by them. Don't hesitate to have a trend analysis performed by those who specialize in this area. The worst thing you can do is *nothing*. If you do not risk, risk will come to you. Many corporate empires are alive and well today because they saw the direction the ecomony was going and began to diversify. If, when people become health conscious, they reduce their consumption of Coca-Cola and start drinking Minute-Maid orange juice, the Coca-Cola company will be none the worse. It markets *both* products.

I believe the same basic rules of risk taking as described earlier apply to financial ventures. You have to have a goal, an objective, and clearly define this objective. Do you want to make a lot of money in a hurry or do you want to play it more conservatively? Most quick-gain risks, such as oil wells or real estate, are quite risky because the odds of success are low. Most long-term gains, such as a savings account, IRA investment, or money-market certificates will realize a high return only on the long haul. What's your goal, a quick kill or a gradual return? The greater the risk, the more caution you should use.

For those who want to own their own business with the promise of high earning at low risk, consider buying into a franchise. Franchising has grown by leaps and bounds, up 9 percent just in the last year. (For more information see *USA Today,* Nov. 8, 1984, p. 68.)

Once you identify your objective, you should apply Rule One: research the risk factors to determine closely what the outcome will be. In business this is called performing a cost/benefit analysis—or trying hard to estimate potential losses versus potential gains. This is relatively easy to do when physical things are being evaluated, but much harder when trying to understand all the complexities of human transactions. Sit down with paper and pencil and list all the pros and cons. But, as you do, remember Rule Two, many risks are hidden. This means *further* research! Dig, dig, dig. If you are investing in a person or business, check the credit rating, check people they do business with, and try to understand their integrity, loyalty, etc. Look at their assets, consider collateral if it's a loan. Look at the length of time they've been in the business. If it's a new business, they still have footprints. How long were they in one place previously? What did they accomplish? What are their professional credentials for the role you may risk of them to perform? Play the devil's advocate. Look for loopholes in the investment scheme. How much does your investment represent of your total worth? Here are some financial risk factors.

- Time necessary to recover initial investment
- Person or business past performance (credit rating)
- Length of time in business
- Need for the service (marketing research)
- Assets of company or person invested in
- Professional credentials of those you risk upon
- Marketing strategy to be used
- Percentage of your total worth investment
- Health of person you invest in
- Manufacturing cost versus retail cost
- Employees opinion of company and those who run the company

Now calculate the likelihood of the events on your list by rating them from one to ten: ten meaning it's almost sure to happen, one that it's highly doubtful. Some items will be easy to rank but others will be tricky. Try to eliminate personal bias and be as objective as possible. Then total the columns. If the benefits outweigh the costs, odds are you are taking a smart risk toward your ultimate goal. But, if costs outweigh benefits, all is not lost.

Ask yourself if you can change anything to bring the costs and benefits into better balance. Be creative. If you personally helped in some area of the risk venture, such as management, marketing, sales, or distribution, would the odds change? If the odds still don't look good, remember Rule Four: Timing is all important, something may work at one time and not another. Maybe the time isn't right. Consider another type of financial venture and use the same technique.

Now for an example from my own life. At one point I needed money to finance one of my adventures. I'd concocted a crazy idea called the Doggie Bag many years earlier while in graduate school. It involved a fast, effective, low-cost way to exterminate fleas. The cost was one-tenth the traditional dip method. It involved walking the dogs into a bag, fitting an adjustable Velcro collar around the dog's neck and zipping the bag closed around the animal. Now, how to get the agent in to kill the fleas? By using

The Doggie Bag®

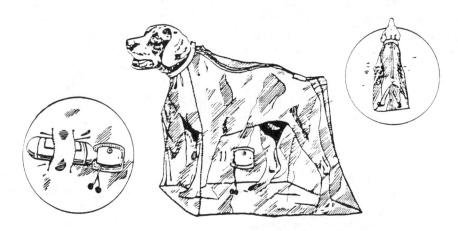

The "Doggie Bag" was a financial risk the author took which paid off. The idea behind the device was to provide a quick, effective low-cost way of automatically eradicating fleas and ticks from the dog's body.

a small cylinder of toxic gas and a puncturing mechanism similar to that which rapidly inflates emergency flotation devices, the bag is rapid inflated with gas.

Interesting as this idea was, nothing had been done to pursue it. Let me now describe how I used the four rules of risk taking to maximize my chances of success.

First, I researched the need for such a device. Conservative estimates were that 2,000 dogs a day in Kansas City received a flea and tick bath at a cost of $12.00 to $20.00. A patent search revealed that several bags had been invented, though none used a totally automatic process of delivering the agent (gas) inside the bag. With the Doggie Bag, as I conceived it, all one need do is pull the rip cord and toxic gas fills the bag.

Before investing any more money, we decided to have one made and try it out. The bag worked beyond my wildest expectations. After testing it on more than 50 dogs we were extremely impressed at its effectiveness. Because it was a do-it-yourself-at-home deflea process and the bag was a one-time purchase, we decided to pursue marketing of the product. I have listed the pros and cons and the subjective value scale that helped in my decision to take this risk.

Pros (Subjective Value)		*Cons (Subjective Value)*	
Make good return on initial investment to be deferred over a six month period	8	Could lose my $500.00 investment	10

Pros (Subjective Value)		Cons (Subjective Value)	
Because of flea epidemic sales apt to be high	8	Patent might not be issued	10
Nothing similar on market to compete with product	7		
No cost to build prototype	9		
TOTAL SUBJECTIVE VALUE	*32*		*20*

Thus, after listing pros and cons (cost/benefits) and using the subjective scale, it seemed the idea was worth the risk. A sizable profit was realized from this venture. I'd researched the risk and the timing seemed right.

In concluding this chapter on risk, I would like to leave you with a story about a patient I had several years ago. He told me that from the time he was thirteen years old, his dream was to make a million dollars before he was forty. He did a lot of risking. He risked financially in the oil business and did very well. But risking financially when the stakes are high can create a very stressful lifestyle. This patient ignored his health, drank and smoked heavily, and of course he was so busy risking in oil he didn't have time for something as trivial as exercise. By the time I saw him, he owned several large oil wells and was worth almost 2.5 million dollars. He was forty-seven and looked sixty. He had severe coronary artery disease and was on twenty-seven different medications. He said he'd give it all away to be pain-free. Think about that. He was superb in analyzing risk factors in the oil business but he ignored risk factors in other areas of his life. The rules of risk taking are simple but they have broad implications. They can help determine your fate, and make life a whole lot easier.

By combining risk factors of each type you can predict your own life expectancy. Start with the number 72 and see how you do.

Personal Data

If you are male, subtract three.

If female, add four.

If you live in an urban area with a population over two million, subtract two.

If you live in a town under 10,000 or on a farm, add two.

If a grandparent lived to 85, add two.

If all four grandparents lived to 80, add six.

If either parent died of a stroke or heart attack before the age of 50, subtract four.

If any parent, brother, or sister under 50 has (or had) cancer or a heart condition, or has had diabetes since childhood, subtract three.

Do you earn over $50,000 a year? Subtract two.

If you finished college, add one. If you have a graduate or professional degree add two more.

If you are 65 or over and still working, add three.

If you live with a spouse or friend, add five. If not, subtract one for every 10 years alone since age 25.

Health Facts

If you work behind a desk, subtract three.

If your work requires regular, heavy physical labor, add three.

If you exercise strenuously (tennis, running, swimming, etc.) five times a week for at least a half hour, add four. Two or three times a week, add two.

If you sleep less than six hours each night, or more than nine, subtract four.

If you sleep seven to eight hours each night, add two.

Are you intense, aggressive, easily angered? Subtract three.

Are you easygoing and relaxed? Add three.

Are you happy? Add one. Unhappy? Subtract two.

Have you had a speeding ticket in the last year? Subtract one.

Do you smoke more than two packs a day? Subtract eight. One to two packs? Subtract six. One-half to one? Subtract three.

Do you drink the equivalent of quart bottle of liquor a day? Subtract one.

Are you overweight by 50 pounds or more? Subtract eight. By 30 to 50 pounds? Subtract four. By 10 to 30 pounds? Subtract two.

If you are a man over 40 and have annual checkups, add two.

If you are a woman and see a gynecologist once a year, add two.

Age Adjustment

If you are between 30 and 40, add two.

If you are between 40 and 50, add three.

If you are between 50 and 70, add four.

If you are over 70, add five.

Add up your score to get your life expectancy at this time. Now compare it to the national average for various ages:

Age Now	Male	Female
0-10	69.8	77.2
11-19	70.3	77.5
20-29	71.2	77.8
30-39	71.3	77.9
40-49	73.5	79.4
50-59	76.1	79.0

Age Now	Male	Female
60-69	80.2	83.6
70-79	85.9	87.7
80-90	90.0	91.1

If you'd like to improve your life expectancy, look over the questions relating to health practices, find those that cost you years, apply wellness behaviors, and you should win in the Monopoly Game of life. Now let's examine why we do the wrong things.

CHAPTER 10
Selected References

Lindsay, Peter H., and Donald Norman. *Problem solving, Decision Making—Decisions in a Social Context,* Chapters 14–16 from Human Information Processing. Academic Press, 1972.

Why People Take Risks

I live in terror. I am afraid of so many things . . . it is a fear of the unknown
. . . and yet, I go ahead and do them anyway, because in making the unknown
known, you become a stronger person, you are better able to deal with life.
—Dr. Joyce Brothers, psychologist and media personality

The race car driver eases himself into the cockpit of his formula race car, preparing for speeds near 200 mph, knowing his life could end in a flash. A teenager goes without lunch, instead putting her quarters into video game machines when defeat is always certain. Phil buys only one brand of soft drink, saving the caps in hopes of winning $100,000. Betty is married, yet she risks dancing with a stranger because she feels a certain attraction to him. Tom will risk all his savings on a sure-fire real estate transaction. All of these people are risk takers, even though the nature of the risks differ.

Some of the reasons why people take risks include:

1. Innate need—the quest for sensation
2. Boredom
3. Challenge and learning experience
4. Addiction
5. Social pressure—the Risky Shift phenomenon
6. Money and fame.

We will examine these reasons in this chapter.

Innate Need—the Quest for Sensation

Although I have chosen to categorize risk-taking motives into six areas, they are *all* related to our needs for stimulation. In this section I want to impress upon you how powerful this need is. It provides the life juice that is the source both of our creativity and of our discontent and destructiveness. It is a biological need common to *all* mammals.

When our basic survival needs for food, drink and warmth are satisfied, we do not simply hibernate until driven into action by the next upswing in our hormonal cycles. Like other mammals, we spend a great deal of time in play and exploration of our physical and social environment. Even the lowly rat will explore a new environment, work to turn lights on and off, and vary the pattern it follows to get to the same place. Curiosity and exploration seem to increase in mammals that are higher up on the evolutionary scale. Who deserves more, you or the rat? Each day has many mazes and we should go in search of the untraveled route from time to time if we want life to remain exciting.

Sensation seeking is a human trait that seems to be genetically encoded. this trait is currently defined as:

> the need for varied, novel, and complex sensations and experiences and the willingness to take physical and social risks for the sake of such experiences.

Dr. Marvin Zukerman, a psychologist from the University of Delaware and author of *Sensation Seeking,* in which this definition appeared, is one of the foremost experts in this area. Through extensive research he has developed a test of sensation-seeking behavior. It has been refined and validated as a true construct of human behavior through extensive research with many subjects over a 17-year period. The test that appears here is somewhat similar to the actual scale and should provide you with a reasonable estimate of where you fall on this dimension of human behavior. Take the test and we'll discuss the implications afterwards.

Test of Sensation-seeking Behavior

DIRECTIONS: Each of the items below contains two choices, A and B. Please write which of the choices most describes your likes or the way you feel. In some cases you may find items in which both choices describe your likes or feelings. In some cases you may find items in which you do not like either choice. In these cases mark the choice you dislike less. It is important you respond to all items with only one choice, A or B. We are interested only in your likes or feelings, not in how others feel about these things or how one is supposed to feel. There are no right or wrong answers as in other kinds of tests. Be frank and give your honest appraisal of yourself.

1. A. I would like a job that requires a lot of traveling.
   B. I would prefer a job in one location.
2. A. I am invigorated by a brisk, cold day.
   B. I can't wait to get indoors on a cold day.
3. A. I get bored seeing the same old faces.
   B. I like the comfortable familiarity of everyday friends.
4. A. I would prefer living in an ideal society in which everyone is safe, secure, and happy.
   B. I would have preferred living in the unsettled days of our history.

5. A. I sometimes like to do things that are a little frightening.
   B. A sensible person avoids activities that are dangerous.
6. A. I would not like to be hypnotized.
   B. I would like to have the experience of being hypnotized.
7. A. The most important goal of life is to live it to the fullest and experience as much as possible.
   B. The most important goal of life is to find peace and happiness.
8. A. I would like to try parachute jumping.
   B. I would never want to try jumping out of a plane, with or without a parachute.
9. A. I enter cold water gradually, giving myself time to get used to it.
   B. I like to dive or jump right in the ocean or a cold pool.
10. A. When I go on vacation, I prefer the comfort of a good room and bed.
    B. When I go on a vacation, I prefer the change of camping out.
11. A. I prefer people who are emotionally expressive even if they are a bit unstable.
    B. I prefer people who are calm and even-tempered.
12. A. A good painting should shock or jolt the senses.
    B. A good painting should give one a feeling of peace and security.
13. A. People who ride motorcycles must have some kind of unconscious need to hurt themselves.
    B. I would like to drive or own a motorcycle.
14. A. If I encountered an extra-terrestrial creature I would approach him or her and attempt to communicate.
    B. If I encountered an extra-terrestrial creature I would not want to make an approach.
15. A. I would work behind a desk every day for $20/hour.
    B. I would work as a charter pilot every day for $5/hour.
16. A. I enjoy a smooth, gentle airline flight.
    B. I like the excitement of bumpy airline flights.
17. A. I think when it comes to sex, variety of partners is the spice of life.
    B. When it comes to sex, one partner is adequate to keep me satisfied and content.
18. A. If someone's opinion is different from my own, I will casually point out the difference.
    B. I am usually inclined to attack someone's point of view if it differs from my own.
19. A. I would like to try speed skiing at 40 mph.
    B. Someone who would try speed skiing at 40 mph is risking serious injury.
20. A. I can't understand why anyone would feel thrill and excitement at the prospect of stealing.
    B. Even though I do not steal I occasionally feel the urge to steal just for the excitement.
21. A. I enjoy breaking fashion, that is, wearing unusual or different clothes or hairdos.
    B. I like to be fashionable, be in style, to look "in."

Scoring: Count one point for each of the following items you have circled: 1A, 2A, 3A, 4B, 5A, 6B, 7A, 8A, 9B, 10B, 11A, 12A, 13B, 14A, 15B, 16B, 17A, 18B, 19A, 20B, 21A. Add up your total and compare it with the norms below.

   1–5   Very low
   6–11   Low
 12–15   Average
 16–18   High
 19–21   Very high

Although the test gives some indication of a person's rating, it is not a highly reliable measure. One reason is, of course, that the test has been abbreviated. Another is that the norms are based largely on the scores of college students who have taken the test. As people get older, their scores on sensation seeking tend to go down.

Readers who would like to take a more precise measure and contribute to Zuckerman's need for normative data may write to him at the Department of Psychology, University of Delaware, Newark, Delaware, 19711. He requests that you send a self-addressed stamped, 8½ x 11 envelope, which he will return with the latest form of his sensation-seeking scale. Mail in the answer sheet with another stamped envelope, and he will send back a complete analysis based on your own age and sex. I suggest you do this in order to see how you do on each of the sub-scales of the actual test. You can learn a lot about your specific needs for stimulation.

My own overall score is 17. The test questions reflect four different ways of expressing sensation-seeking behavior: thrill and adventure seeking, experience seeking, disinhibition, and boredom susceptibility. For example, all those questions that relate to high-risk sports indicate a desire for thrill and adventure seeking. I score the maximum on this dimension since I enjoy adventure sports and the challenges and learning opportunities they provide.

If you are a high sensation seeker, you probably have many adventurous tastes—from an eagerness to try risky sports such as skydiving to a desire for a variety in sexual partners.

As a group, high sensation seekers rate the dangers of such activities lower than those who generally seek less stimulation. Even when high and low sensation seekers appraise the risk in the same way; the high sensation seekers contemplate the activity with more pleasure than anxiety, while the low sensation seekers experience nothing *but* anxiety.

Translating this to everyday life, high sensation seekers are more likely to pursue risk-taking activities of either a positive *or* negative nature, as discussed in the last chapter. In his research on sensation seeking, Dr. Zuckerman found they are more likely to smoke, drink excessively, take drugs, violate speed limits, and engage in heterosexual experiences (the riskier the better). They often pursue occupations like police work, firefighting, flying, or, at the very least, occupations that involve lots of people contact, which they find stimulating. Because they do not appraise fear to the same extent as the low sensation seeker, they tend to prefer higher odds and gamble in various other forms much more frequently. In terms of the wellness model in section I, this factor is what ultimately leads to their self-destruction. The difference between playing and gambling is a matter of controlling the odds. You are playing when the odds are weighted in your favor. You are gambling when the odds are weighted against you. Keep this in mind, because if you gamble, the odds will eventually catch up with you.

As I said, I'm a high sensation seeker. My needs for adventure and challenge are extremely high. To some degree, this was a motive for doing the feats described earlier in the book. However, I like to be in control, and I take positive risks, ones which further my growth on the wellness continuum.

Some questions in the full-scale test relate to alcohol abuse, drug abuse, or people abuse since many high sensation seekers find middle-class life tedious and seek escape in heavy drinking, partying, gambling, and a variety of sexual partners. But this mode of sensation seeking ultimately leads you down a dead-end street. Such activities have no character-building attributes and will ruin your health, as I point out in this book. I know they seem enjoyable, but high-level wellness offers better alternatives. Try to understand the impact of what's happening to you when you choose these forms of stimulation. You choose them because they create a temporary increase in arousal. And we need increases in arousal level just as certainly as we need air, water, food, and shelter. All of us have this strong biological need. If we can't get it one way, we'll get it another. Young autistic children will rock back and forth on elbows and knees to create this needed stimulation. There are alternatives, other ways to get your "fix," which are natural. But our modern lifestyle has made negative risk taking much easier, cheaper, and more accessible. One dollar and one minute can buy you a caffeine, nicotine, alcohol, and sugar high. But positive risk substitutes last longer, they help you achieve your loftiest dreams in life.

Many health/wellness professionals would do well to understand this principle. It doesn't suffice merely to tell a person to stop drinking, smoking, using marijuana, overeating, etc. You must be prepared to provide reasonable alternatives. People aren't computers. They are active stimulus seekers. This is one reason people who quit smoking often gain weight. They simply substitute one form of stimulation for another.

We've come so far in the last hundred years but we may lose our perspective if we don't re-focus our risk-taking behaviors. Be exploratory, be curious, seek out the positive risks until you find one you can sink your teeth into and then, *Go for it!*

The illustration on page 151 shows the pleasure areas of the human brain. We all have a biologically determined level of stimulation for staying well. The secret is, "How much?"

The Pleasure Areas Of The Human Brain

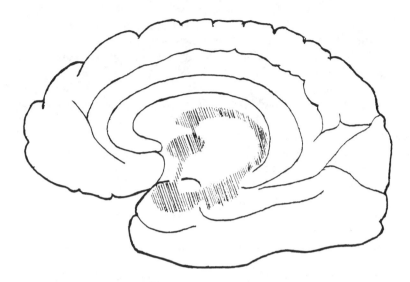

The shaded areas in the illustration represent the pleasure areas of the brain as seen from a medial view of the right hemisphere. These primary pleasure areas are; the hypothalamus, the hippocampus, the fornix, the septum, and the amygdala. When animals have been trained to press a lever and deliver shock via an electrode implanted within these areas, they will stimulate themselves repeatedly, even up to 5,000 times an hour. If permitted, this behavior may continue to exhaustion, even taking precedence over food.

One scientist even believes evolution has progressed not so much to favor greater size and strength, but to allow the organism to derive more pleasure from the environment. Greater size and strength merely happened coincidently in order to increase the pleasure-seeking opportunities.

Listed below are sports which high and low sensation seekers seem to prefer in order to meet their needs for stimulation.

Activities High SS Prefer	*Activities Low SS Prefer*
Downhill skiing	Tennis
Martial Arts	Golf
Waterskiing	Bowling
Sport parachuting	Walking
Hang-gliding	Bicycling
Mountain and rock climbing	Swimming
Fast dancing (rock and roll)	Slow Dancing (ballroom)
Hunting	Nature trips
Paraplaning	

Other sports like jogging, racquetball, and scuba diving may interest both groups; however, research has shown that their approaches will be qualitatively different. High sensation seekers, for example, are more daring, since they do not appraise the risk as high and thus tend to be more injury-prone. Being more exploratory, high sensation seekers may engage in risky sports for longer durations. In test situations involving scuba diving, they will remain underwater longer on their first dive or dive deeper if a fixed time limit is set.

Since high sensation seekers tend to be more dominant and aggressive, they will probably be much more competitive than will low sensation seekers. Finally, high sensation seekers seem better adapted to handling situations requiring danger, speed, and vertigo. This may be one reason they enjoy high-risk sports and high-risk occupations.

Lest you think high sensation seekers are crazy because they are attracted to high-risk sports, let me quote Dr. Zuckerman, addressing the 1980 International Congress of Applied Psychology.

> We do not have to postulate unconscious death wishes or masculine protests to explain their desire for adventure, and excitement. These desires, more characteristic of some than others, are part of our biological heritage. They are part of the source of our exploratory and creative activity as well as destructive behaviors in crime and war. High risk sports, along with travel, art, music, sex, and social stimulation, can meet sensation seeking needs even if work cannot. Unfortunately, for a civilization that cannot provide adventure and stimulation for the young which is socially acceptable, crime and drugs (negative risks) may meet their needs.

The value of a Columbus or a Lindbergh to a society is incalculable. We must wonder if, denied the opportunity to go exploring, these great men might have wound up as cocaine addicts.

Many psychologists believe that criminals are a product of bad environments, that is, they come from underprivileged homes. Dr. Stanley Samenow, a criminal psychologist who has studied criminals for fourteen years and written *Inside The Criminal Mind,* disagrees. They commit crimes because they enjoy it, he asserts:

> Murder is exciting. Robbery is exhilarating. Criminals commit crimes not because they come from underprivileged homes, take drugs or watch a lot of violence on TV but because they like to.

Like most criminal psychologists, he used to think criminals were simply products of bad environments. But, after hundreds of interviews, Dr. Samenow now believes the sensation-seeking motive explains much of their behavior

> In my daily clinical experience I find that criminals create crime because they like it. Crime is their oxygen. It gives them a kick like nothing else.

When asked to explain why most of the people in prison were poor and black, he answered,

> What the statistics reflect is that our system of justice falls far short of being just. The well heeled and influential, with their access to competent legal counsel, are often likely to avoid winding up behind bars.

Our innate need to be exploratory has been somewhat checked in our advancement toward a more civilized state. We seem to have upset the natural balance of man interacting with his environment. As Desmond Morris, writing in *The Human Zoo* explains:

> As a species, we originally have been intensely active and exploratory in connection with our special survival demands. The difficult role our hunting ancestors had to play insisted on it. Now, with the environment extensively under control, we are still saddled with our ancient system of high activity-high curiousity. Although we have reached a stage where we could easily afford to lie back and rest more often and more lengthily, we simply cannot do it. Instead, we are forced to pursue the stimulus struggle. Since this is a new pursuit for us, we are not yet very expert performers and we are constantly going too far or not far enough. Then, as soon as we feel ourselves becoming over-stimulated and overactive or understimulated and underactive, we veer away from the one painful extreme or the other and indulge in actions that tend to bring us back to the happy medium of optimum stimulation and optimum activity. The successful ones hold a steady center course: the rest of us swing back and forth on either side of it.

Morris believes a lot of our present-day distress, inappropriate risk taking, and abnormal sexual behaviors can be traced to overly complex society with its overcrowding, confined, and artificial constraints. Again, in his own words,

> Under normal conditions, in their natural habitats, wild animals do not stimulate themselves, masturbate, attack their offspring, develop stomach ulcers, become fetishists, suffer from obesity, form homosexual pair-bonds, or commit murder. Among city dwellers needless to say, all these things occur. Does this, then, reveal a basic difference between the human species and other animals? At first glance it seems to do so. But this is deceptive. Other animals do behave in these ways under certain circumstances, namely when they are confined in the unnatural conditions of captivity. The zoo animal in a cage exhibits all these abnormalities that we know so well from our human companions. Clearly, then, the city is not a concrete jungle, it is a human zoo. The comparison we must take is not between the city-dweller and the wild animal, but between the city-dweller and the captive animal. The modern human animal is no longer living in conditions natural for his species. Trapped, not by a zoo collector, but by his own brainy brilliance, he has set himself up in a huge, restless menagerie where he is in constant danger of cracking under the strain. Despite the pressures, however, the benefits are

great. The zoo world, like a gigantic parent, protects its inmates: food, drink, shelter, hygiene and medical care are provided; basic problems of survival are reduced to a minimum. There is time to spare. How this time is used in a non-human zoo varies, of course, from species to species. Some animals quietly relax and doze in the sun; others find prolonged inactivity increasingly difficult to accept. If you're an inmate of a human zoo, you inevitably belong to this second category. Having an essentially exploratory, inventive brain, you will not be able to relax for very long. You'll be driven on and on in more and more elaborate activities. You'll investigate, organize and create and, in the end, you'll have plunged yourself deeper still into an even more captive zoo world. With each new complexity, you'll find yourself one more step removed from your natural tribal state the state in which your ancestors existed for a million years.

What this means, is that we need to make a *conscious* effort to avoid all the entrapments and negative risks made so convenient by the human zoo: cigarettes, "adult 25-cent movies", marijuana, junk foods, and other self-defeating stimulants. It means we need to pursue sports, fitness, and mental activities that fulfill our exploratory and inventive natures while also enhancing our physical, social, and spiritual growth. In short, we need to be a better animal.

Boredom

The term boredom is used to describe the negative feeling produced by a monotonous environment. Distress can result not only from having too much to do, but also from *having too little to do,* or doing the same task repetitiously. Psychologists call this situation *stimulus monotony.* Examples abound in our society where the daily work routine is highly regimented, highly predictable from day to day, and fails to maintain a high state of interest and arousal. I recall a job I had as a high school student working evenings unloading a conveyor belt. It got so I could do this half asleep. This was very distressful to me. I felt like a robot. It required no thought whatsoever.

Many of the filing clerks and secretaries I've interviewed in different companies say they can almost perform their entire eight-hour work day with eyes closed. As Dr. Zuckerman stated, "People will get their stimulation in one form or another." And risk taking usually fulfills this need. Witness the explosive interest in many high-risk sports, such as mountain climbing, hang gliding, skiing, and wind surfing in recent years.

Boredom is a very potent force in driving people to take risks. The best way to think of risk taking is to think of it as playing a game. In fact, game theory is often used to describe gambling and other forms of risk-taking behavior. What are the essential components of a game? Here they are.

- Games involve a series of moves from a number of possible choices.
- Moves are made by you, by your opponents, and, to some degree, by chance.
- Some moves are open, some hidden, some made with incomplete information.
- Strategies are used to trick the opposition.
- There is a payoff along the way or at the end, depending upon the odds.
- Personal values and preferences will be a factor in your decision to maximize gains and minimize losses.

Again, when faced with a risk-taking decision, ask yourself the question, am I playing or am I gambling? Sometimes, in order to counter boredom, the player or participant in the game of risk taking doesn't really care whether he wins or loses. He simply enjoys being in the action. How often have you bet on a football game not so much to win money but to enhance the excitement of the game? As Clark Hudak, Director of the Washington Center for Pathological Gambling in College Park, Maryland puts it:

> They can't stop . . . they become addicted to the action of gambling. Win or lose becomes secondary to the feelings they derive from being in the action. . . . Boredom is characteristic of the pathological gambling personality. The quest for stimulation, challenge, excitement often ends only with the action, the escape.

"Being in the action" is fine as long as you don't run out of money, or your health, or both. Gamblers Anonymous is an organization that can provide help for those with this disorder.

Television commericals often employ the boredom strategy to lure you to their products or services. They offer excitement, good times, and fellowship. They appeal to your need for self-esteem, your need for sexual companionship, and even your sense of virility or femininity. The list of products is endless: alcohol, drugs, cars, clothes, candy, soft drinks, shaving cream, furniture, and chewing tobacco. Vance Packard's best selling book, *The Hidden Persuaders,* provides more information on this topic.

One car commercial states: "Feel the sense of excitement it gives you as it hugs tight corners and accelerates from 0 to 50 in only four seconds."

One manufacturer of shaving cream dramatically illustrates how it won't stop a locomotive, only a voluptuous brunette. The strategies or moves are well concealed. They hire movie stars, professional athletes, or grandparent figures to sway your decision making. The "Marlboro Country" theme helped R.J. Reynolds sell a lot of cigarettes. It has AC-TION, roping cattle, riding fast horses, taming the wild west. Now they will even sell you western wear. Gee, now you can lie back in your recliner (with boots and cowhide vest) and conjure up stimulating images while you blow smoke signals across the living room range.

I used to have this terrible problem. I didn't have any friends. And I didn't know what the problem was. But, then one night I was watching TV and I figured it out. The very next morning I ran down to my neighborhood convenience store and bought a Dr. Pepper. I held it up as high as I could, ran outside, and starting dancing and singing, "I'm a Pepper, I'm a Pepper, wouldn't you like to be a Pepper too?" People started gathering around me like crazy. It was simply amazing. And just in case there might be some hostile people in the crowd, I had some M&M's to pass out. Man, I was IN.

Even something as simple as breakfast involves risk taking. Eggs and bacon, or skim milk and cereal? Coffee or milk? Butter or margarine on the toast? Soft drink or orange juice? The payoff they claim is "feeling great," or "gives you energy," or "makes you feel like a new person," or "all the neighbors will envy you."

Many psychologists agree that extramarital sex occurs because of boredom. The excitement of "the chase" can offer much for a marriage bankrupt of romance and the unpredictable.

Boredom and the Roller Coaster Syndrome

A bored society will not only tend to drink more, smoke more, and abuse drugs, but will engage in other more exotic and socially acceptable forms of thrill seeking behaviors. Much of this takes place in amusement parks, the king of attractions being the roller coaster, an American tradition since 1884.

A roller coaster, for all its thrills and excitement may simply be termed a *controlled fear*. All over the United States every day thousands of people buckle up so they can scream for several minutes as they feel their body accelerate down 120-foot drops, sense the centrifugal force throw their internal organs outward on fierce curves, and roll upside down through corkscrew turns.

The heyday of the roller coasters was in the 1920's when as many as 2,000 were scattered around the country. Motion pictures were not widely available, television and video games were not accessible, and the impact of the Industrial Revolution created a work force that sought relief from the monotony of assembly lines and regimentation. Such relief was to be found in the excitement generated by the notable Crystal Beach Cyclone Coaster in Buffalo, the Tornado in Coney Island, and the Rye Playland Aeroplane in upstate New York. TV and the automobile soon offered alternative forms of stimulation and the economic hardships of the thirties left roller coasters standing deserted, like remnants of a ghost town after the Gold Rush. By the late seventies only 200 existed, although this has drastically changed in recent years with a tremendous increase in such rides.

So, what is a roller coaster designed to do? To provide the greatest possible thrill at the lowest possible risk, to fool the many bodily reflexes and neurological control mechanisms nature designed to keep us oriented and balanced in three dimensional space. Many of these are located in the inner ear compartments. Rapid shifting of fluid in these compartments caused by acceleration or rotation stimulates neuromuscular activity throughout the body and increases arousal levels in higher brain centers. The end result is a more alert, more aware animal. Such stimulation can be quite exhilarating indeed. It can also be very therapeutic, as I'll explain later.

I dare say not many of you would get on a roller coaster (Or any amusement park ride for that matter) if you actually believed for one moment that your life was in peril. What you seek is the *perception of fear without the reality*. This is a controlled fear. On the contrary, many bad habits, like smoking or drugs represent *the reality of danger without the perception*. Yes, the body can fool the mind, and the mind can fool the body.

I often use the roller coaster analogy in describing my own stunts and extreme sports since what I also sought was a controlled fear, or *rational risk taking,* which I'll define shortly. Like the roller coaster engineers and manufacturers, I'd researched and eliminated the actual dangers.

How safe are roller coasters? The Consumer Products Safety Commission estimates that 3 billion people attended carnivals and amusement parks in 1980 (up 22 percent from 1970). Reported injuries severe enough to require emergency treatment at a hospital numbered between 6,000 and 8,000 and most were soft-tissue injuries like abrasions, sprains, and lacerations. After reviewing the data and case histories I found that in many cases where death or injury occurred, the rider was attempting to add to the thrill and excitement by standing up, not fastening seat belts, rocking the cab, or otherwise ignoring the normal safety precautions.

Compared to a roller coaster, a merry-go-round doesn't seem very intense, right? Well the percentage of injuries on merry-go-rounds was almost *twice* that of roller coasters.

High-intensity activities like roller coasters and other amusement park rides produce the elevated arousal and stimulation many people need to offset feelings of boredom. Although potentially very therapeutic, access to such activities is limited by financial and geographical factors. This is why I advocate high-intensity sports (kayaking, skiing, rock climbing, and ultradistance running). They can be pursued often. In a world bereft of physical challenges, controlled stress is still the best antidote to boredom there is. As Dr. George Mandler, a psychology professor at the University of California at San Diego, observes:

You know where a roller coaster is going to go, you have every reason to believe that it is going to get there at the end . . . there is no feeling of helplessness, no disorganization, and under those conditions arousal produces positive affects.

Seek out the natural environmental challenges. Beware the "roller coaster syndrome"—extreme danger without the perception. Drinking and driving may be fun, but the ride may end abruptly. Boredom can be a potent force for taking big risks.

Personal Challenge and Learning

A lot of people want and will seek greater challenges in order to probe their deeper resources. One of the most creative examples of this is the philosophy of the Outward Bound program that originated in Colorado, the brainchild of Kurt Hahn, a German educator. It originally began as a training school in survival skills for young seamen, designed to teach them self-reliance, confidence, conditioning, and bonding with each other. These skills were necessary to the "will to survive." They were taught to take risks, because successful risk-taking produces an attitude of hardiness, that is, that all things can be overcome. Eventually, the program expanded to the general public. Outward Bound has worked with the courts to take wayward children, drug abusers, and juvenile delinquents and offer them positive risks instead of crime and other forms of negative risk-taking behaviors.

By substituting real-life adventures full of challenge and controlled risk from activities like rappelling, white-water rafting, and mountain climbing, the wayward youths are able to learn many positive character-building traits under the supervision of qualified leaders: teamwork, empathy for others, outdoor wilderness skills, conversation, perseverance, first aid, and the importance of physical fitness in order to achieve goals. They also learn to solve problems in a particular situation and analyze risks.

Outward Bound has grown enormously and now has programs in seven states. Many of these wilderness schools have now adopted their programs for executives, teaching lessons in teamwork and self-exploration. The theory underlying the executive course is that

> people learn their own capabilities and limitations far better when they are faced with immediate physical tasks that require cooperative decision making.

The manager of employee development for a large aerospace and construction materials manufacturer said of the program, "the employees came away with the thought that if they put their minds to a task, they can do virtually anything."

Another comment also sums up the experience very well;

I learned that taking risks is what life is all about. With alcohol I risked dying. So why not risk becoming honest with myself and get in touch with reality? Why not risk living?

Outward Bound has been in existence for some 30 years. During that time 13 of the 70,000 students have met with fatal accidents, most by drowning. Outward Bound emphasizes safety procedures but knows there is a strong element of risk. Still, the challenge is the lure and many thousands of people have come away from their experience more confident, more fit, more aware of their strengths and limitations. I believe one paragraph from their brochure sums up their philosophy:

> An Outward Bound course is not easy. It's not meant to be. Physically strenuous and mentally challenging, it is personal achievement in the face of doubt, accomplishing tasks you thought were impossible, learning to expect more of yourself than you dared before.

Outward Bound will send you a conditioning program several months prior to your participation to help ensure that you are fit to meet the required challenges, much as I did prior to my risky adventures. I wish we had more schools of "experiential learning" like Outward Bound. Fortunately, there is a trend in this direction at the university level. Risk taking is part of the curriculum for students enrolled in the Adams State College—Mesa College cooperative guidance and counseling Master's Degree program. Dr. John Holmes, director of the program, explains:

> Counseling is a series of risk taking situations. Counselors must learn to take risks and understand how a client feels when they enter the foreign environment of a counseling session.

In one of their projects, students must scale a wall blindfolded and rely on others to break their fall. One student remarked:

> I learned more about myself in three and a half hours at Adams State College than I did in four years of undergraduate study at another school.

This program is called Rational Risk Taking. To quote from the course description:

> Participation in high risk activities should be based on evaluation of personal skills. When an individual preceives risk inappropriately or evaluates personal skill inaccurately, the chance of physical injury is increased. This same perception process is true of other areas of life (misperceiving risk or incorrectly evaluating personal skills). If either of these conditions occur, no possibility exists for rational risk taking.

Rational risk taking is what I call the ability to perceive risk factors and eliminate them. It results in the student's being able to make more efficient and effective choices in *any* area of life. Only in this way, Dr. Holmes believes, will students reap the long-range benefits of risk experiences, in other words, achieve their personal and career goals. This is indeed a creative and constructive approach to risk taking. There are so many character traits such risk-taking courses can teach us, including trust, self-confidence, and enhanced problem-solving ability.

Prescott College (Prescott, Arizona) is another school (fully accredited) where experimental learning in the wilderness combined with classroom lectures provides a unique learning environment. Risk-taking experiences provide a philosophical framework to help bridge the gap between school and the real world.

Dr. Sol Rosenthal, a physician and biochemist who has devoted a great deal of his life to researching risk taking, has defined what he calls the *risk exercise,* also called RE. It differs from the common concept of risk taking in that it is measured. He also feels we need challenges but they should be controlled challenges. The primary assumption of RE is that the risk taker has the skills to match or overcome the risk. Otherwise, says Dr. Rosenthal, you have a maniac doing something with no other predictable outcome except terror or despair. This concept of developing the skills to match the risk level implies forethought or evaluation of the risk factors and each person's ability and skill to deal with them.

The real thrill of the RE response, Dr. Rosenthal feels, comes when the risk tests the skills of the risk taker. This represents the challenge. As he puts it, "It takes him up to the far frontiers of his skills, but it should not take him mindlessly beyond it."

Dr. Rosenthal also prescribes RE for many of his patients because of its therapeutic value. Some of the positive benefits he sees in measured risk taking include:

1. A feeling of having achieved more of your potential as a human being, of feeling deeply fulfilled and having a much greater expectancy of life.
2. Feeling more keenly aware of the world around you and developing what may be called an X-ray texture of the world, the ability vividly to see answers to some current life problems.
3. Unlike the negative risk takers who become separated from reality via drugs or alcohol, the positive risk taker is more reality based. He is better able to sift among the many sensations and mental clutter and set meaningful life priorities.
4. Measured risk taking (positive risk taking, as I call it) produces an exhilaration, even euphoria that lasts much longer than mind-altering drugs. There are no side effects either.

Dr. Donald Vest, a psychologist at Washburn University who has taught a course called "The Psychology of Risk Taking and Sensation-Seeking Behavior," sees risk taking as a necessary challenge for many people because it serves as "stress reduction through stress in-duction." When asked why so many people are seeking the pursuit of marathons, triathlons, hot-air ballooning, and other risky activities, Dr. Vest stated:

> People are engaging in these sports because their current pursuits, whether vocational or recreational haven't offered enough intensity, involvement, or activation of mind and body. More dangerous activities force a person to pay attention to just what they are doing. They focus within a narrow range and simply must pay attention. You can't worry about the office when you concentrate on getting your feet set right on the rock you're climbing. It's kind of a forced escape, but one with positive consequences like emotional release and physical conditioning.

Yes, positive risk taking can be fun but remember: *Be sure your skill level is matched to the risk!* Many accidents occur every year because some fool ignored all the safety precautions, forgot to manage the risk factors. It's natural for people to upgrade the risk as they upgrade their skills. The skier seeks out more demanding slopes, the surfer goes to bigger waves, the rock climber to steeper faces, and the jogger to longer runs.

Whether you are a low or a high sensation seeker, the RE response is not absolute. There is a positive risk exercise for everybody. Sailing may seem very risky for some people (the low sensation seeker), while not risky at all for the high sensation seeker. Regardless, proper safety precautions should be used to eliminate the risk factors. This means wearing a flotation device, learning to sail in favorable weather, and having a suitable craft. Horseback riding was a risk exercise prescribed by Dr. Rosenthal for some handicapped children. The results of confronting a challenge like this were enormous. The children gained much self-confidence, and had a lot of fun too.

Addiction

Many substances are highly addictive, most notably tobacco, caffeine, alcohol, sugar, and drugs. Even addiction to one's own biochemicals can occur.

In 1954, James Olds, a psychologist, discovered that if electrodes were implanted in an area of the brain called the limbic system, the animal would self-stimulate, once taught to do so by pressing a lever. Hundreds of studies have since verified such brain areas which produce sensations of pleasure (see illustration earlier in this chapter). Some of the most remarkable studies have demonstrated that an animal will continue to self-stimulate to death, ignoring food, water, and even a female in heat in order to stimulate this pleasure area of the brain.

There are substances found in the brain called endorphins. These chemicals produce a feeling of euphoria in response to a physical stress like strenuous exercise. This fact has been used to explain the addiction that drives many runners to push beyond their limits and develop stress fractures. They simply lose control and self-destruct. This lack of self-control thus makes further running a negative risk activity. These endorphins are also released during psychological states of fear and pronounced stress and seem to work in opposition to adrenalin-triggered responses such as fast heart rate and elevated blood pressure. They slow respiration, lower blood pressure, and calm the nervous system. Research has shown that high sensation seekers have lower levels of endorphins in the pleasure areas of their brain. This means they may *need higher risks or stresses to produce the same feeling of euphoria.*

Quite often, after completing my risk activities, I've noticed this pronounced sense of euphoria, often lasting 24-48 hours, and probably caused by the release of these substances. There is always this feeling of tremendous power and control over the events of my life. I seem to know with certainty how to deal with many ongoing situations. This rarely happens when I run, although I have observed this effect after a hard distance race. Thus, high-risk activities can become quite addictive if we aren't careful. I've met some skydivers who go without eating in order to finance their skydiving habits. These endorphins in helping us to cope may prove to be even more powerful in their effects than sex. Certainly, many subjective reports seem to lead to this conclusion. Monoamine oxidase, a chemical found in the brain that is responsible for transmitting nerve impulses to the pleasure centers, has also been found to be lower in high sensation seekers, *requiring more intense stimulation to produce feelings of pleasure.*

Video computer games may illustrate another risk-taking activity that is highly addictive. There have been several media reports of young people committing crimes to support their habit. Several heart attacks while playing have also been reported. Besides losing his money, the player may also lose his life.

Dr. Robert Eliot, a noted cardiologist at Nebraska University Medical Center, has classified some people as hot reactors, meaning they show dramatic increases in blood pressure, heart rate, and certain stress hormones. In many cases, the systolic blood pressure increased 60mm Hg., a dangerous elevation. Heart rate can also increase dramatically. The whole "fight or flight" response is triggered (see chapter 9), and the heart rate/blood pressure may be much higher than running on a treadmill. Dr. Eliot says, "That's like drag racing with the brakes on."

One of Dr. Eliot's subjects was thought to be a "cold reactor" until a woman was sent in to compete with him, sending his diastolic pressure to 102. Guess what? The woman's blood pressure went off the chart at 188/120. Fortunately, most people are cold reactors; I'm one of them.

No one knows for sure whether video games cause endorphins to be released, but we do know these games are highly addictive. Dr. Eliot states that "For at least ⅓ of the people who play, the payoff is the powerful internal kick from playing."

Social Pressure—The Risky Shift Phenomenon

The risky-shift phenomenon has been well documented by social psychologists for many years and probably is one of the major factors contributing to negative risk taking.

The risky-shift phenomenon is best explained by describing a typical research experiment. When subjects were brought into a room one at a time and asked to handle a snake (which had been rendered harmless, though subjects did not know it), few were willing to do so. However, when brought together as a group and asked to do so, more than half the subjects would handle the snake. What is it about the group that increased the subject's willingness to take this risk? Some researchers believe it is a disinhibition effect produced by numbers. There seems to be security in the fact that others will join in. This diffuses responsibility among group members, reducing the fear level.

The most recent research indicates that the cultural values of a society will determine to a large degree whether there is a shift in either the high risk direction or toward the conservative direction when a risky decision is required. In the United States, for example, where our culture places high value on risk taking, a group of people would be more apt to take higher risks than the individual person. This may explain why gangs or groups of youths commit crimes, steal cars, or sell drugs when any one member, left to himself, might not.

Whatever the mechanism of change toward greater risk, one thing is sure. There is a reduction in the perceived fear level. Just by way of example, The Surgeon General's Office has mandated the dangerous effects of cigarette smoking for many years now. And yet, in a national survey, 25 percent of the respondents said they didn't know smoking was bad for their health.

Money and Fame

Stuntmen are actually professional risk takers who do it for a living. They take risk seriously and carefully plan each stunt. Because of television shows like *That's Incredible* and *Games People Play*, there is a whole new breed of amateurs trying extremely dangerous stunts to gain instant fame. Both of these shows have had their share of mishaps with people being crippled for life. Some of these shows pay the performer substantial sums of money to film their stunts. Deran Sarafian, associate producer of stunts for the NBC show, *Games People Play*, asks:

Where do we draw the line? Who's a legitimate stuntman, an expert at minimizing the risk and who is not? What's entertaining and what's merely toying with the human life for profit? Where are the guidelines?

The guidelines are to be found in the performer's motives. What does jumping over a speeding car demonstrate? I can't understand televising some form of extreme risk taking without trying to communicate an educational idea. Risk to demonstrate human potential in terms of endurance, strength, courage to overcome handicaps, etc., Yes. Risk, just to give the viewer an adrenalin rush, No! THOSE should be the guidelines. Risk for benefiting others' growth, okay. Risk for risk's sake? Why not just turn the gladiators and the lions loose?

Before ending this chapter, I'd like to mention briefly some new forms of sensation and accompany this with my observations and opinions on the safety of these new activities.

New Forms of Sensation Seeking

The *Fly-Away*   This is a new way to experience the thrills of skydiving without having to jump out of an airplane. It is a DC-3 engine enclosed within a silo, which creates a wind tunnel effect. You crawl onto a grid from side benches and (while wearing jumpsuits for added lift) fly-away, that is rise into the air. A few of these are now found at amusement parks, and keep looking for one near you. The popularity is growing since everyone wants to experience flying. No data is available on their safety.

The *ParaPlane*   Half airplane, half parachute, this device is ingenious both in its effects and in its safety. It can be folded into the trunk of your car, set up in 30 minutes, doesn't require a pilot's license, and Presto, you're airborne. Unlike hang gliders, which require hangars, more expense, troublesome assembly, and more training, the ParaPlane is relatively safe since you are already under a parachute should the motor stop. It's rather inexpensive too. It comes pre-assembled. Contact the ParaPlane Corporation, 5801 Magnolia Avenue, Pennsauken, New Jersey (609-663-2234).

Recumbent cycles   These are like bicycles but are much closer to the ground with the rider lying in a semireclining position. The low center of gravity creates a lot more feel of the road and they also have more speed on level ground because of the reduced air drag. The three-wheeled versions are a blast but be careful. Their low-slung profile is also a safety hazard if proper visibility flags, lights, etc. aren't added. Contact the Human Powered Vehicle Association in Seal Beach, CA at 213-420-9817.

Pedal-powered one-man skull   Made by Knapp Sea Saber in Healdsburg, California, this machine is raw speed on the water. It weighs only 50 pounds, can go 12 mph, is 21 feet long, and is a great way to add to an aerobic program. It can easily outrun any four-man skull team and is simply a pedal powered propeller which scoots you through the water. An inexpensive kit can be obtained to convert any small boat to pedal power.

Triathlons and their Cousins

A triathlon usually combines running, swimming, and bicycling. I believe the phenominal growth rate of this sport represents a population hungry for challenge and the variety of the natural landscape. In fact, perhaps more than any other single sports event, triathlons offer the promise of overall fitness of mind, body, and spirit. Endurance, strength, and flexibility are gained if one trains properly and most triathlons fulfill the requirement for spiritual growth (chapter 13) if a genuine commitment is made. The positive risks are summarized below.

1. Life becomes more exciting. The combination of three separate sports adds more variety and enthusiasm to ones life. Boredom becomes less likely (if not eliminated altogether).
2. Addiction to one sport and the tendency to overtrain in search of more and more stimulation is reduced. This is because your energies are channeled across three different sports and the transitions between those sports which is a major factor in both training and competing. If an injury should occur, merely focus on the other two until you can resume the third one.
3. Overall fitness balance is achieved since endurance, strength, flexibility, and skill development are outcomes of such involvment.

Some triathlons substitute kayaking for swimming, and quadrathlons include climbing. Biathlon events (running and cycling) are also increasing in frequency. Cyclo-cross combines cycling and running over rough terrain while carrying the bicycle. I predict more versions of triathlons and quadrathlons will germinate over the next 10 years. I learned one version in the Marine Corps Boot Camp at Parris Island, South Carolina. We ran five miles, climbed several 20-foot ropes, swang by rope from a high platform (over water), splashed in and swam for home. Health promoters, let your imaginations go. For information on Triathlons near you, contact 619-565-9416.

The Survival Game

A revival of earlier times and a game of rapidly growing proportions, this is an adult version of cowboys-and-Indians or "capture the flag." It is a living PAC-Man game played with guns. the idea is to capture the other team's flag and return it to "home base" without getting shot. The gun is CO_2 powered and shoots gelatin capsules filled with yellow paint. A "kill" occurs whenever someone is marked with a splat of paint. The battle zone is typically a 20-acre section of rented farmland, selected for its topographical features, i.e. rocks and lots of trees to hide behind, tall grass, a few ditches or ravines, and if you're real lucky, a decrepit shack or shed of some kind. Of course, you wear camouflaged clothing and grease your face with earth tones, the better to kill without being killed.

Now, if you're like me, you value human life and find war disgusting, then the idea of stalking another human being for pure adventure seems sick, perverted and (to borrow a quote from Shakespeare) "Between the acting of a dreadful thing and the first motion, all the interim is like a hideous dream."

But wait now! There's more than meets the eye. As in all else, opinions devoid of experience are as light to a blind man. Could such a game promote wellness? Perhaps it does indeed.

After some three hours of playing, I found that "Survival" was a tremendous amount of fun at a nominal cost ($15.00-$21.00). You see, no one really takes it seriously, all players maintain a sense of humor, yet know that cunning strategy, quick decision making, teamwork, skill, and fast reactions help achieve success. In a word, adults leave their status symbols behind when the horn sounds the game, become as children once again, for in this game everyone is equal. Also, a "flow experience" occurs and (as we will see later) this is stress management at its best.

Does this game release violent inhibitions—create people more ready to explode? It doesn't; just the opposite happens. It siphons off the aggressions and anxieties of the real world. Better to participate in an outdoor game of mind/body involvement than watching games on a television set where overgrown gladiators purposefully attempt to inflict damage on other human beings in the name of play.

In almost two years since its inception, not one single incidence of violence has been reported. Dr. Lester Mann, a psychologist from Penn State University who studied the game, found "no evidence to indicate that it creates aggression in people." He endorses "Survival" as a healthy outlet for aggression. Some companies are using it to enhance employee relationships. As in any sport, if you follow the rules, like wearing goggles to protect the eyes, it's highly unlikely anything more than a slight sting from a pellet will occur—unless, of course (like me), you go diving through the brush and land in a patch of thorns.

And what about physical fitness? My heart rate, I found, reached 156 beats per minute and remained there for twenty minutes during the first game, sufficient to provide some cardiovascular benefits. Such is always not the case. The games can end quickly, the result of too many players on both teams. Fewer players, a large battleground, less time between games, or other rule variations designed to promote more endurance would enhance the potential fitness contribution. Lionell Atwill's admonition (author of the Survival Manual) "Forget basketball, hockey, tennis, and golf" is just not correct, for a game played once or twice a week does not suffice in the real survival game of life. If this becomes your only avenue for fitness, my advice would be to use it as an individual sport, or no more than three people on a team. Game kits (include guns, ammo, goggles, etc.) can be purchased from most survival game dealers. Tracts of land at the city's outskirts can be found so that you're not bound to an official game field or committed to a "green fee." This would allow for more frequent, longer playing games and greatly enhanced physical fitness.

Environmentalists take note: I believe the Survival Game contributes much more to mental health and wellness in general than does the more traditional sport of hunting various forms of wildlife. Why? Two reasons:

1. As a potential source of fitness and stress management it's much more practical and *nothing gets killed.*
2. Game birds can't shoot back!

So, I'm suggesting you give this a whirl. You'll probably meet some new friends, have a fair workout, and enjoy a diversion from a boring lifestyle. Who knows, maybe you'll even leave some of your primitive self behind and go home more relaxed than when you came.

For more information on Survival Dealers near you, contact 1-800-225-PLAY.

Computerized Exercise Equipment

I predict this trend will revolutionize the boredom and drudgery of indoor exercises such as stationary cycling. Digital feedback of distance covered, speed, heart rate, calories burned, or simulated courses like that seen on the popular Lifecycle make such exercises much more stimulating. Someday you'll put a cassette in your VCR, plug your stationery bike into a computerized module which interfaces with the VCR and cycle through glorious Colorado Mountains or Oregon Evergreens on the screen while the resistance automatically changes to fit the terrain you're watching. Keep watching, it's coming.

And if you want to climb to the top of the World Trade Center in your living room, the Stairmaster by Tri-Tech Inc. will let you do so with a computerized display that keeps you motivated with printouts and a built in cassette player. So what next?

How about memory telephones built into your computerized exercise equipment. When you reach a desired calorie burn rate, it automatically dials your sweetheart. If you fall below the criterion . . . whoops (a recording) . . . "Sorry, sir, you've been disconnected. Please pedal a little faster."

CHAPTER 11
Selected References

Atwill, Lionel. *The Official Survival Game*. Simon & Schuster, 1984.

Heyman, S. "Sport and the Sensation Seeking Motive." *Psychological Foundations of Sport and Exercise*, (ed.) John Silva and R. Weinberg, 1983.

Morris, Desmond. *The Stimulus Struggle*, Chapter 6 from The Human Zoo. Dell Publishing Company, 1969.

Skow, John. "Risking It All—The Spirit of Adventure Is Alive and Well." *Time,* Aug. 29, 1983.

Zuckerman, Marvin. "A Biological Theory of Sensation Seeking." from M. Zuckerman, (ed.). *Biological Bases of Sensation Seeking, Impulsivity and Anxiety*, Lawrence Erlbaum Assoc., 1983.

CHAPTER 12
Risk for a Heroic Goal

What we now need to discover in the social realm is the moral equivalent of war; something heroic that will speak to man as universally as war does, and yet will be as compatible with their spiritual selves as war has proved incompatible

—William James

The heroic goal is something anyone can strive for. But not everyone will. That's what makes it heroic, a special high to reach, lofty pinnacle where you can set your sights and, with the motivation of this chapter, rise to fame.

You probably won't make the front page of your local newspaper, but then you won't really care. You didn't do it for that. The fame you achieve is probably limited to your family, friends, and co-workers. But still you are famous. Because for the rest of your life, no matter who you meet or where you meet them, you can tell them that you went beyond. You can tell them you soared beyond mediocrity, went exploring, left the human zoo, if only for awhile. You did something few others dared to do.

Perhaps what really makes you a hero more than anything else is that you become a change agent. By your inspirational example you can significantly influence the lives of numerous other people and the effect becomes multiplied many times over. Your example makes you a wellness ambassador and this more than anything else is what makes the heroic goal so important. By your example you create a ripple effect . . . others help others!

The heroic goal probably won't decrease your risk of heart disease beyond the limits described in chapter 9. But, humans are more than a circulatory system or a walking anatomy textbook; they are spiritual beings capable of reflection, abstraction, and continued growth (which comes from taking risks). They are also, in highly technological societies, capable of suffering from chronic boredom. As evangelist Dr. Robert Schuller of the Crystal Cathedral in Garden Grove, California reminds us:

Desires [for worthwhile goals] are important because they release a force

we call passion. The passion releases you from boredom. We now know that
next to a loss of self-esteem, boredom is the basic emotion behind alcoholism
and drug experimentation. Boredom is probably the number one reason for
experimental, antisocial, and un-Christian behavior, normally called S-I-N.

The heroic goal may save your soul, it is an experiment in "possibility
thinking."

The Anatomy of Heroism

There are three stages to heroism.
Stage 1. Preparing   This means doing "something suitable to the character of a hero." Examples are:

1. Giving up cigarette smoking
2. Giving up refined sugar and other "junk food"
3. Starting an exercise program
4. Losing 15 pounds
5. Any change which improves your wellness

Stage 2. Committing   This involves setting a long-range goal that requires determination and courage to complete.
Stage 3. Completing   This involves actually achieving that goal. It
means following through with your plans and overcoming the obstacles.
When this has been done, you're a hero. Now for some examples.
At Washburn University I taught a course for those who work with
the handicapped. The motto I gave my students was "all things are possible." We explored this belief among handicapped people and I believe
we can learn a lot from their examples.

Some Incredible Heroes

Ron Gilstrap of Conroe, Texas, waterskis—without skis—barefooted.
He not only waterskis barefooted, he does this with *only one leg*. Ron lost
his right leg in a serious motorcycle crash in 1972. Says Ron:

> For a year and a half I really felt sorry for myself. I began drinking heavily
> and was just wasting my life away. I went from 180 pounds to 225 pounds
> with just one leg. I had to find something that would make my life worth living.
> . . . Waterskiing really changed my life. I was kind of a bum before the accident
> but learning to ski in conjunction with the loss of a limb gave me a new
> perspective on life. I look at things differently now. In order to survive, you
> must fight back.

Ron first did something heroic. He gave up his drinking. Then he
committed himself to a heroic goal. Now he is a hero.

Don Perry of Albuquerque, New Mexico, scuba dives, rappels, swims, and waterskis. A lot for one person to handle? Consider this: Don was born without one arm and one leg. Don says, "I don't consider myself any different from anyone else. My philosophy has always been—just do it."

Harry Cordellos competed, and completed the 1980 World Ironman Triathlon in Kallua Kona, Hawaii, an event consisting of a 2.4 mile ocean swim, a 112-mile bicycle race, and a 26.2-mile marathon run in 16 hours. Harry also waterskis barefooted. Not bad, especially for someone who is totally blind! He has also run the Boston Marathon, canoes, kayaks, ice skates, and cross-country skis. Harry is a hero.

Norman Croucher climbs mountains. At 40 years of age he conquered the 21,509-foot Himalayan peak White Needle. It was only the fourth time in history this peak had been scaled. He also scaled the Jungfrau, the Eiger, and the Matterhorn. He also hiked 900 miles across England. Yet Norman Croucher has no legs. He was run over by a train while drunk. Says Norman, "The more serious risk is not losing your life, but wasting it."

And who will forget Terry Fox's 3,339-mile run across the landscape of Canada, his "Marathon of Hope" to raise money for cancer research. Terry lost his right leg to cancer a year earlier. Cancer spread to his lungs and finally forced him to stop. Said Terry, "It beat my body, but never my spirit, I pushed myself to the limit." Terry was awarded the Order of Canada—the highest medal a Canadian civilian can receive. Terry is a hero. And how about the seven former heart attack patients who entered the 1971 Boston Marathon with their coach and cardiologist, Dr. Terry Kavanaugh. They all finished. They are heroes.

Perhaps you're thinking, "Those were all young people. I'm too old. I could never do anything that difficult". Well then, consider the following case history.

Eula Weaver, at eighty years of age, was a walking pharmacy; she took aspirin for arthritis; Pro-Banthine for her GI tract; Arlidrin as a vasodilator; Digoxin for the heart; nitroglycerine for her angina; Aldomet, Esidrex, and K-lyte for her high blood pressure. She wore gloves in the summer because her circulation was so bad. She could walk no farther than 50 feet from her home, after which she had to be carried back. After a long history of heart trouble that included frequent angina, a heart attack, and congestive heart failure, she finally became bedridden, She was spoon fed, and had to be dressed. She could easily have given up.

Under constant supervision, she began a program of low-intensity, frequent walking combined with a very low fat diet (the Pritikin Diet— almost identical to what I call the Primitive Diet.)

Two years later, she was walking three miles and riding ten miles a day on her stationary cycle. She also did some light jogging. By this time she was drug free.

In 1975 she entered the National Senior Olympics in Irvine, California. Five years later, at ninety, she had accumulated ten gold medals and a plaque for her performances in the half-mile and mile events.

Finally, there is Hulda Crooks, an eighty-seven year old woman from Albuquerque, New Mexico. Hulda has climbed Mount McKinley twenty-one times. She never began climbing until she reached age sixty-six. Eula and Hulda are heroes. So why not you?

Be Your Own Hero

You *can* be heroic too. All you have to do is initiate some positive health action. Risk some change. Give up your present comfort zone and go in search of the better you. Then set a heroic goal. This can be any physical accomplishment that demands endurance and commitment in order to prepare for and complete. In the process you will come to a better realization of yourself, strengthen your inner resources, and achieve a depth of satisfaction not known before. Some examples are:

- Marathon
- Triathlon—perhaps even a minitriathlon
- Extended cross-country ski trip
- 500-mile bicycle trip (for those over 50, a 100-miler).
- Marathon swim
- Mountain climb or difficult rock climb
- Long hiking trip of extended distance (100 miles) over rough terrain
- Extended canoe or kayak journey

The important thing is that you go the distance, overcome obstacles of mind and body. In our soft world it is easy to slide from day to day, never testing ourselves, never knowing the ecstasy of self-discovery. Going through the three stages to becoming a hero and dealing with the risks to achieve that goal will give your life new meaning. An example of this change is reflected in the following letter:

Dear Dr. Crookse:

This letter is in response to the recent *Kansas City Star* article called "Feat was Part of a Greater Philosophy". I greatly admire what you are doing - the points you made in the article have had considerable validity for me. I am a 34 year old high school biology teacher. I enjoy my work, but financial rewards just aren't there.

About a year ago, I started long distance running and my philosphy of life has undergone some dramatic changes. For the first time, I am goal setting (something I'd stopped doing). Currently I am training for the New York City Marathon in October with a goal of 3½ hours (A noble goal considering I'm not a natural athlete.) My previous interest in material possessions and feeling sorry for myself because I wasn't making much money has diminished. My running has not only made me physically healthier, but has made me mentally tougher. I also like myself better now.

The point is, what you say WORKS. It has been happening to me and now I'm glad someone is communicating this in words. I look forward to your coming book.

Best wishes,
Rick Gould

Rick did complete the marathon in the time he set for himself. Rick is a hero.

I am at odds with many of my professional colleagues, because I do not think there are very many people who will give up bad habits in order to live four or five years longer. Statistics will not work. They sit on your tongue for awhile, like castor oil that's good for you if you can swallow it, then gets spit out. They have no personal relevance. People need a better reason than that. They need a stronger, more viable motive. I believe the cleansing process of the heroic goal fulfills this need. As Dr. Don Ardell, author of *14 Days to a Wellness Lifestyle*, states:

> I have come to suspect that heroic acts often provide the mental strength needed to engage, sustain, and escalate a wellness lifestyle.

Payoffs of Risking For a Heroic Goal

Whenever you take something away from an individual upon which he has had a long-standing dependency, you need to replace it with something else that will provide a substitute satisfaction. Again, the heroic goal provides this. The payoffs for risking to achieve a heroic goal are many:

Personal responsibility is instilled. You succeed or stall on your own merits. You quickly come to realize that the goal cannot be had if you continue to smoke, drink heavily, and abuse your body in other ways. Therefore, you learn that the Spartan lifestyle will get you to your heroic goal.

Nutritional awareness As Dr. George Sheehan says, The runner doesn't care about health, he cares about performance. Health is just a stage he goes through in order to get there.

Yes, anyone seeking maximum performance from his or her body soon learns the do's and don'ts of nutrition, that a diet high in natural fruits, vegetables, and whole grains is vastly superior to the typical, highly processed, low-fiber diet. The many hours of training are lessons in optimal vitamin/mineral intake. As you pursue your heroic goal, you will begin to eat better because food will be thought of not only as a means to curb your hunger but as a form of fuel! You will not want to put low octane fuel in your sleek Maserati body.

You learn to control stress.   Time priorities must be established to prevent energy drains. Visualization and relaxation skills (deep breathing, meditation, etc.) assist you in preparing for the various stresses of competition, harder training, and good sleep patterns.

Greater self-awareness   Present limits are constantly being extended. Self-esteem continues to escalate as the heroic goal is approached. Confidence grows and spills over into other areas of your life. In reaching new limits you may become aware of new forms of consciousness, described by Charles Lindberg during his historic flight from New York to Paris.

> For unreasonable periods I seem divorced from my body as though I were an awareness spreading out through space, over the earth and into the heavens, unhampered by time or substance, free from the gravitation that binds men to heavy human problems of the world. My body requires no attention. It's not hungry. It is neither warm nor cold. This essential consciousness needs no body for its travels. It needs no plane, no engine, no instruments; only the release from flesh which the circumstances I've gone through make possible.

Lindberg was an avid walker, walking up to five miles a day while thinking over the problems he would encounter and how he would resolve them in order to achieve his dream.

Abundance of energy   If you use common sense training rules and stay in control, you will find that, as you become more and more fit, your energy reserves increase many times over. Listen to your inner feelings, do not become rigid in adhering to a schedule. Maintain a flexible attitude. Stay calm. Condition yourself and when things feel good, go for it. When your energy level continues to go up, you know you are doing things right.

Character traits improve   You cannot become a hero without first becoming a better person. The Spartan life teaches us lessons like perseverance, dedication, and commitment. When I had the opportunity to visit with many triathletes at the World Ironman Triathlon, in Kona, Hawaii, I was very impressed by their set of values. It had cost many of them lost income, but the "purification" of this achievement gained through countless hours of training had given them a lot more—a sense of deep personal pride and inner glory money cannot buy. Money cannot buy heroism. It is earned during many lonely hours of toil and sacrifice.

Regarding this last benefit, pursuing a heroic goal to its completion, I would like to borrow a few lines from the late and great Percy W. Cerutty, coach of many world class athletes and world record holders.

> In a word, there is no impossible barrier that cannot be broken through and which can separate forever a thoughtful man from his reasonable objec-

tives. . . . Character and personality rests on an intelligent application of our gifts and a recognition of our shortcomings, together with the determination to develop the former and overcome the latter. . . . Success then, is based in both thought and action. With either factor absent, or in too little content, great success is as a dream without substance.

I tend to ignore the big name sports heroes, if indeed they are! I cannot call such people heroes who promote the junk food industry. Real heroes cannot be bought off. Rather, I call *you* the hero, the silent hero who risks leaving mediocrity and all its false gods behind and goes in search of the heroic goal. Let me list the essential factors of that goal.

Description of a Heroic Goal

First and foremost, it must be something which requires you to experience a sort of crisis in your life, that is, a goal so difficult that you must take certain risks and give up the "easy life." You may risk some friendships, probably some income, and perhaps some injuries. The latter can be easily avoided with common-sense training principles as described in chapter 13.

It must be an event in which you extend yourself, *for* yourself. Because of this I recommend that much of your training time be in solitude, for only then will you truly get to know your deeper self. Indian folklore often required young men to go off into the woods for protracted periods, in order to "Hear the song of the wind, the echo of footsteps, and sharpen the wisdom" they had been taught. If you "recruit" someone else with a similar goal they may carry you along and you will not achieve the strength that comes from self-reliance.

The activity should be one that develops endurance, although ideally you will also attempt to develop some muscle strength and flexibility in the name of balanced fitness.

There should be a final climactic event or endpoint against which to measure your progress. However, success is not measured by time so much as by the completion of the event for its own sake. No one has failed who completes a marathon.

The event or heroic goal should take at least six months of preparation. If it is achieved in less time than this, you have cheated yourself because the degree of difficulty was not severe enough to build the character traits discussed.

Selection of Your Heroic Goal

Answer the following questions even if right now you do not plan to become a hero. You may change your mind. I will gently guide you through the thought process.

GOAL ANALYSIS

What events or ideas do I have that I fantasize doing someday that now seem impossible?

_____

_____

Examples   Marathon, ride to Chicago on a bike (500 miles), swim 10 miles non-stop.

Now, divide this heroic event or activity into one-fourth of the amount stated above.

_____

Examples   Run 6 miles non-stop, cycle 125 miles, swim 2.5 miles.

Now, for 3 minutes close your eyes and see yourself completing it. Fix it in your mind, imagine how you look, feel, act. Were you happy, proud, high, ecstatic? Write down how you looked or felt.

_____

_____

Examples   Looked 15 lbs. lighter, felt very proud of myself, had the look of a real champion.

Describe the risks you will take to achieve only this one-fourth journey to your heroic goal.

_____

_____

Examples   Less time with my wife, time for my work, cost of the equipment, impatient with those who are mediocre.

Now, list the benefits you may realize (social, mental, personal, and emotional).

_____

_____

Examples   Better condition, more confident, less bored, more self-satisfied, more outgoing.

How long will it take you to reach this modest goal enroute to the heroic one?

_____

Example   2 months

See, when you break it down into manageable parts, it does not seem quite as hard. I suggest you keep the heroic goal tucked away in the back of your mind and focus on the modest one for several weeks. Get checked over first for safety purposes. After a few weeks, reassess your larger goals, but go after the smaller one with all your enthusiasm. When I began each of my adventures (some do not qualify as heroic goals) I could not initially see myself doing them. But each step up the ladder was a learning process and my confidence grew as I went. Usually, only about one month before each event did I really begin to believe I could succeed. The courage comes in trying, making the effort. When Terry Fox began the pursuit of this heroic goal, it was all he could do to run a quarter-mile.

Risks of Pursuing a Heroic Goal

There are a number of risks which you should be aware of once you have reached Stage 2, actually training for your heroic goal. I will list these risks, but only to prepare you if they occur. Any lofty goal always has a number of risks, but in positive risk taking (chapter 10) the payoffs always far outnumber the risks since they foster personal growth.

Addiction   You risk becoming overzealous and trying to do too much too soon. This is very common. Many endurance athletes have become addicted to the high—euphoria of endurance training only to progress much faster than the recommended training load (10 percent increase per week in training volume) and develop stress fractures. My question to these people is, "Is the activity controlling you or are you controlling it?" One of the lessons of sport is self-control. Everyone has hormones called endorphins which, once released, can have highly addictive influences. They have even been compared to psychedelic drugs in their effect.

Separation From Others   Your success in pursuing your heroic goal may make old friends act strangely or seem hostile. To put this behavior in the proper perspective, remember the words of Pulitzer Prize-winning journalist Thomas Powers, who was quoted as saying:

> The winners in life don't forget their old friends, the old friends withdraw. They back away not because of what you've done, but because you remind them of what they haven't done.

Water does indeed seek its own level.

False Expectations   Be sure you are setting your goal for yourself, not for competitive purposes. Otherwise, as happens in any successful endeavor, people around you will expect repeat performances, want you to go farther, faster, higher. And, if you're not constantly in touch with your true motives, you may fall into this trap.

Loss of Income   Right now this may seem a very real risk. However, what you may delightfully find is that you become more efficient at work. Also, as your values change and you measure everything less in dollars and cents, you may find you are quite content with less money and more self-satisfaction. As pollster Daniel Yankelovich reports in his book *New Rules,* in the past, success meant improvement of one's social position (more money and more status). Today, he reports, 66 percent of Americans consider success to mean improvement of the self. I'm not saying money isn't nice, I'm just saying what's much more rewarding in the long haul is the "warm toasty feeling of knowing you've challenged and won". Psychologist Rollo May once wrote, "To the extent that we fulfill our potentialities, we experience the profoundest joy to which the human being is heir." I sincerely hope each one of you can experience this joy.

There you are. You should by now have the incentive to go in search of your larger self. Remember, a trip of 100 miles begins with one small step, giving up a bad habit, beginning tomorrow. There will be days when you can't seem to get going or the world seems to have conspired against you. But, if you take the time to sit down and make a short-medium-and long-range plan, you are on your way.

As we close this chapter, I will leave you with what I have discovered to be the greatest benefit of setting and following through with a heroic goal.

Somehow, an emotional crisis often occurred within the one to two month period prior to each of these risky events. But, because my focus was on preparation for the event, and because of the challenge it represented, I didn't come unglued. It provided such a strong sense of purpose, *it acted as a kind of buffer against other life crises.* I could put the crisis in better perspective, especially after completing my goal. When you near the completion of your heroic goal you'll understand this feeling. It's as though you have shed your old skin along with all the old fears and insecurities and grown by one quantum leap. You become mentally and physically stronger. You risked. You won!

Once you set a heroic goal and are ardently working toward that goal, your score on every area of the Risk Taking Questionnaire in Chapter 1 will improve. Your life will take on more meaning. You will avoid negative risk taking like the plague.

Before planning your heroic goal be sure to read the next chapter. It will help you over some of the pitfalls. Remember, the heroic goal is a wellness challenge that can help you achieve peak performance in every area of your life. At the very least, it will dispel your boredom and rekindle your zest for life.

CHAPTER 13
Safety Rules For Heroes

I advocate that you risk for a heroic goal. By becoming more aware of possible pitfalls you can better achieve that goal. No doubt I'll be attacked by the conservative element—in fact, I expect it, because this is not a book on how to be mediocre. If you want to achieve peak performance you'll have to take risks. Remember the Wellness Continuum? The greater the risk, the greater the rewards can be. Follow the information in this chapter and we can help quiet the critics.

The Risks

The first step is a *safety check*. We live in a society where wellness is the exception rather than the rule. Several studies have shown that in any random sample of middle-aged population, as many as 10 to 15 percent will show signs or symptoms of heart disease. That is why proper medical screening is a good idea.

Between 1979 and 1984, sixteen people in the United States died while running, including Jim Fixx. Thirteen of them had known heart problems prior to the fatal attack.

A medical study of runners published two years ago statistically pegged the risks of running: one death per year for every 7,620 runners, or one death per 396,000 hours of running. If we assume a very slow average jogging speed of 7 mph, then we have one death per every 2,772,000 miles, making jogging one of the safest forms of transportation known to man. A lot more people croak at their desks than die from running. In fact, the most common precipitant of heart attacks is straining during a bowel movement!

Use the accompanying diagram to help you decide what form of clearance you need, especially if you opt for the heroic goal.

For your medical check, try to find a physician with an avid *interest in sports* and fitness, ideally, one who runs and pursues the Spartan life. Check with your local running clubs; they usually know who these physicians are. This person will encourage you and serve as an invaluable

Safety-Proof Yourself

Use the diagram below to determine whether you need to be screened or not. Follow the appropriate arrows.

Primary Risk Factors (PRF)

Smoking History —————————————— Yes — — ┐
                                        — No ┐ │
High Blood Pressure ———————————— Yes ┤ — │
                                    — No ┐ │
High Blood Cholesterol ————————— Yes ┤ — │
                                  — No ┐ │
Symptoms of Heart Disease ————— Yes ┤ — │ *Need Stress EKG*
                                  — No ┘

                          Under 35 | Over 35

┌─────────────────────────┐
│ No Screen Needed   │
│ Be sure to follow safety│
│ guidelines to insure   │
│ goal attainment.   │   *Secondary Risk Factors (SRF)*
└─────────────────────────┘

Family History Heart Disease

Overweight > 10% Normal

Physically Inactive

Under Great Stress

┌──────────┐
│ CONSIDER │
│ STRESS   │ ─ Yes ─ TWO OR MORE PRESENT
│ EKG   │   No
└──────────┘

┌────────────────────────┐
│ Annual Check of   │
│ Blood Chemistry Needed │
│ to reassess PRF   │
│ This vital step will   │
│ insure your safety and │
│ success.   │
└────────────────────────┘

resource in the event some mishap occurs despite your efforts to avoid them. *The Sportsmedicine Book,* by Gabe Mirkin, M.D., is a highly recommended resource.

Next, if you suspect a *structural weakness* in your foot—a very vulnerable area for those engaged in weight-bearing activities—by all means see a podiatrist and consider the use of orthotics, a type of device used to balance the foot forces during impact. This single preliminary step might save you lots of misery on down the road.

First of all, however, get a *good pair of shoes.* Avoid the $9.95 shoe. The Brooks Vantage is a good shoe for beginners, but for those who are 175 lbs. or more, or who plan to cover a lot of miles, I highly recommend the Nike Air-Soles. Studies have shown that red blood cells can rupture very easily because of the excessive jolt from poor shoes and crushing of red blood cells circulating through the feet. Since red blood cells carry oxygen, their loss could decrease your oxygen uptake or endurance potential. Some experts believe this destruction in red blood cells explains the curious finding that runners often suffer from iron deficiency. Also, creatinine phosphokinase, an enzyme liberated in response to muscle tissue injury, is much higher after a standard workout in shoes with poor shock absorption than a shoe of the quality found in the Nike Air-Soles. To put this fact in perspective, what it means is that your recovery rate from a running workout will be much faster with good shoes than with the cheap, poor quality shoe. If you already have a cheap shoe, the use of Sorbithane inserts ($14.00), will help immensely in reducing road shocks.

Now to dampen your enthusiasm—but only for awhile. Get up and go *look at yourself* in a full-length mirror. If you have clothes on, strip down to your undies. Take a long look at yourself and ask if you like what you see. Be completely honest. No fair turning the lights down. While gazing at yourself, close your eyes and imagine yourself when you were eighteen.

Did you like what you saw? Come on, confess. You aren't the same allstar who used to tear up the track or zip up and down a basketball court. If you find a big red "S" emblazoned on a skin-tight blue suit, then you can forget anything else I have to say. Please give me a call, though, I always knew you were out there. I wanted to believe in Superman. Otherwise, if you had a sagging middle and looked like someone was slowly deflating you, heed this advice. Do not expect to go out and get in great shape within two weeks. In fact, a good rule of thumb is to allow two weeks of buildup for every six months you've been inactive. For example, if you've been inactive for two years, you'll need to allow two months to get back in shape. This is called the progression principle.

One estimate states that nearly 20 million people in this country are injured in sports activities each year. Most of these injuries involve muscles, tendons, and ligaments. You need to strengthen the chassis before you overhaul the engine.

You'll progress toward your heroic goal much more easily by increasing your training volume (load) only 10 to 12 percent from week to week where the activity is weight-bearing, as in running. You can increase it 15 percent from week to week if the activity is nonweight bearing, as cycling or swimming. If miles are not the unit of measurement, use minutes or city blocks; in the case of swimming, use pool laps. In rowing, strokes/min will suffice.

Exercise your heart the way you brush your teeth—to build up, you should exercise at least five days per week. I know there are a lot of experts who say three days per week is sufficient. They tell you this because they're afraid you won't do it otherwise and they want to make it easy on you. I want to make it hard on you, but hard while teaching you self-control. How many things in life have you really valued that came easy? Not many, right? You valued what you had to work hard for. Do you think you'd keep brushing your teeth if your dentist told you three times a week was sufficient? Heck, no. That's less than 50 percent of the time. You don't build habits doing something less than 50 percent of the time. I want you to develop the habit of daily exercise to the point where you feel guilty if you miss a day, like you do when your teeth are yucko.

I once met a guy who developed the greatest motivational tool known, his dog. It all started when he took the dog out for a stroll so Rover could go to the bathroom. Rover never quite got his bladder emptied, though. Once in the house, the owner went right to bed. Well, good ol' Rover didn't want a spanking so he wouldn't let his owner go to sleep until the job was completed. The owner, enjoying the night air, decided to go for a long walk, during which time he gave Rover doggie treats because he was so proud of his behavior. This happened for several weeks. Finally, the guy couldn't go to bed if Rover missed his walk. He tried in vain to bribe Rover with a handful of treats. Now, who trained whom, did the owner train Rover, or was it the other way around? Consider training a feline. It may save your life. The message is: five days a week. This is the *frequency principle*.

Your body is like your car; it needs a *break-in period*. If you bought a new car and paid $6,000 for it would you get in it and drive at speeds of 100 mph the first few days? I hope not. You probably wouldn't have any valves left. The same principle applies to your body. When you've been inactive for a long time, you have to break it in gently. This means for several weeks keep your heart rate at 60 percent of its maximum. Then, for another few weeks you can go to 70 percent of its maximum. Beyond that, 80 percent of maximum is allowable. Use the chart below as a guide.

Pulse Beats/Minute

AGE	60% MAX*	70% MAX*	80% MAX*	90% MAX*
20-30	118	140	156	176
30-40	114	135	152	170
40-50	108	126	144	162

AGE	60% MAX*	70% MAX*	80% MAX*	90% MAX*
50-60	102	119	136	153
60-70	99	116	132	149

Take your pulse for 12 seconds and multiply by 5. This will give you beats/min.

Now for the *human factor*. As I have stated elsewhere, human beings need stimulation in one form or another. I seriously doubt if any of you will not feel an occasional "urge to surge," especially you high sensation seekers. This is okay. It is the seasoning, the salt and pepper, that breaks the routine, monotony, and regimentation of your workout. The Swedish do this and call it *Fartlek* or "speed play." You can surge but adhere to the time limits given below for the first few months.

Progression	Surge Time (in seconds)	No. of Surges/Workout
First 3 weeks	10	2–4
Second 3 weeks	20	3–5
Third 3 weeks	30	4–6
Fourth 3 weeks	45	5–7

Follow these heart rate limits and you will be using the *intensity principle*. This principle will help prevent many of the soft-tissue injuries so common to aspiring heroes. This principle somewhat serves as a guide to whether you should walk or jog. It depends on whatever form is necessary to produce the recommended heart rates.

The battery needs to build a charge. Your muscles, like a car battery, will store energy in the form of glucose. But, in order to increase their ability to store greater and greater amounts, your endurance must be built up gradually. The best way to accomplish this is with the *duration principle*. This is the time spent per each exercise session. If you elect to pursue the heroic goal this could involve up 2 to 3 hours/day. You don't have this kind of time? Yes you do. We all do. It's a matter of priorities. You spend that much time watching TV, carousing, and inspecting refrigerator shelves. If busy lawyers, physicians, and other people do it, you can. You are a blue-collar worker? You need this more than anyone because you are the prime target for the sickness industries and you are more prone to suffer chronic boredom. Your income doesn't allow for exotic forms of positive risk taking, so you're extremely vulnerable to the negative kinds. The heroic goal can be your salvation. Time limits are listed below:

Progression	Duration (in minutes)
First 2 weeks	8-10
Next 3-5 weeks	10-15
Next 6-8 weeks	15-20

Progression	Duration (in minutes)
Next 9-10	20-30
Keep Going!	30 +

Okay, so more than 20 to 30 minutes three times a week won't necessarily reduce your risk of heart disease. Who really does it for that reason anyway? I don't. I've met a few people who do. Most do it for the extra energy it gives them, for the relaxation it provides. Well, the more you exercise (duration), the more energy you'll have, and that means feeling more alive!!! It often means feeling a greater sense of *spirituality*. Reducing heart disease is just the frosting on the cake.

Duration is much more important than intensity (speed), both in terms of weight-loss effectiveness, lowering blood fats, and building up the energy stores in your muscles. Don't hesitate to stop 2 to 3 minutes occasionally to enjoy the passing fragrance of a flower, or some other roadside pleasure. Such rest intervals will actually allow you to cover a greater distance and burn more calories. Annabel Marsh, aged 61, and Caroline Merrill, aged 42, trained for their run across the United States by running and walking several times a day until they could cover the 30 miles per day necessary to successfully complete the trip. Hats off to two heroes.

Racket sports like tennis and racquetball are great fun and a super way to socialize. They can also complement your journey to the heroic goal. Notice that I said, "complement". Injuries to soft tissue are high in these sports because of the rapid stop-and-go, stop-and-go action of the game. Racquetball is a great conditioner if you play often enough. The problem is, most people don't. Raquetball or tennis will not suffice for heroic goals because they don't meet the criteria listed. But use them to replace a regular workout from time to time. Tennis is great fun but too often the tempo of the game is so casual little endurance is developed. Low sensation seekers may be quite appeased and satisfied with this as their sole form of exercise. If they are able to be guided by their inner voice and score well on the Life Risk Questionnaire, then what more can we ask? The heroic goal is not for everyone.

Maintain a *sense of balance* in your program. Incorporate strength and flexibility training into your conditioning program. All running or all cycling or all of any one sport is narrow in scope. Dr. Gabe Mirkin says when you start to get an injury, switch immediately to another sport which uses different muscle groups so the injury can heal without your losing any endurance. Bob Anderson's illustrated book, *Stretching,* by Runners World Publication, is highly recommended for all those who seek heroic goals. Proper stretching can reduce the likelihood of injuries.

Primitive man probably engaged from childhood in many activities like running, swimming, ceremonial dancing (of a most vigorous nature for an hour or more during which time he often mimicked animals he wished to kill). Thus, he was never really "out of shape." It's doubtful he ever experienced injuries related to poor strength or flexibility. Balance is the key.

Women may have *special problems* when pursuing heroic goals. Some evidence indicates females have a greater problem with calcium retention when involved in ultradistance running, thus increasing the likelihood they may suffer fractures from decreased bone density. This is especially true in post-menopausal women because of lowered estrogen levels (estrogen aids calcium absorption.) Thus, they may wish to monitor their intake of calcium to be sure it is at least 1200–1500 mg. per day. I would also suggest avoiding diet colas since such high-phosphate drinks tend to leach calcium from the body, further increasing the likelihood of a low calcium state.

A glass of milk contains 300 mg. calcium, and brewer's yeast is also high in calcium. Women who don't drink milk should consider taking a 1000 mg. supplement with iron daily. Iron is another mineral many female endurance athletes score low on.

Women may also be more predisposed to shin splints because of the wider angle of the tibia in relationship to the pelvis. Careful attention to training principles, good shoes, use of Sorbithane inserts, and avoiding concrete as much as possible in the first few months of training should reduce this possibility.

Several recent studies indicate women may stop menstruating when they launch into heroic efforts requiring tremendous investments of time and energy. Such findings, however, have been very inconsistent. One explanation may be the fact that, as most gynecologists know, the onset of any sudden stress or emotional disturbance can upset the delicate balance of female physiology that regulates such functions. As long as a woman is having fun, gives her body the necessary time to adapt, doesn't become overcompetitive (the heroic goal emphasizes competing against oneself more than another person), and eats wisely, she should not encounter this problem. If she does start to skip periods, the best advice is to consult a gynecologist.

Incorporate easy/hard days into your workouts. This assists adaptation to increasingly longer workouts and adds a lot of variety. Tom Osler's system works very well: One day each week do 30 percent of weekly total, two days do 15 percent of weekly total, two days do 10 percent of weekly total and two days 5 percent of total.

Always precede your workout with at least *5 minutes of slow activity* that mimics the intended activity. This is called *specific warmup*. Everyone tells you to do this but few give you reasons why. Here are a few good reasons for doing so.

- When muscle temperatures are raised slowly to their optimal point, muscles contract more efficiently. This happens because there is less viscosity (or resistance) to movement of the tiny fiber strands within the muscle bed. Transmission of nerve impulses is also faster after warmup, enhancing coordination.

- Blood vessels in the muscles dilate (expand), which helps deliver more blood and oxygen to improve the chemical reactions that take place in the muscle cells.

- Warm-up time allows the fluid in the various joint spaces to circulate more, in effect, lubricating the joint surfaces better to reduce wear and tear.

- Slowly stretching the elastic components (like tendons and ligaments) increases their *strain threshold,* the point at which they will actually begin to tear apart. The older one is, the more important this injury-reducing factor becomes.

- Perhaps most important, it allows a time wherein to mentally adjust to the actual activity itself, thereby decreasing the perception of effort, maybe even allowing us to go longer than we otherwise would have. Dilation of vessels in the brain is quite likely the mechanism by which this happens.

Likewise, a cool-down period is also extremely important. If one stops too suddenly, pooling of blood in the extremities can cause faintness, dizziness, and other dangerous situations. For example, recent research has shown that the incidence of abnormal heart rhythms (skipped beats) can occur because the body interprets the pooling of blood as shock and releases large amounts of norepinephrine in the blood. This chemical can trigger life-threatening irregularities in the heart's rhythm. Again, a 5-minute cool-down period should suffice.

Anyone who pursues a heroic goal will probably have to confront *climatic extremes.* The *Sportsmedicine Book* by Dr. Mirkin also provides guidance here. One factor, *superhydration* is extremely important in hot, humid weather. That is, always drink more water than your thirst dictates, since thirst always lags behind actual physiological needs. Eight ounces of moderately cold water every 20 minutes during hard exercise in hot weather should prevent any heat related disorders. Runners—take a lesson from bikers and carry water with you in plastic containers strapped about the waist. Avoid salt tablets and tea (a diuretic), which only speeds the loss of fluid from the body.

The following signs and symptoms indicate *overtraining.* I'm big on teaching would-be superstars to self-monitor in order to foster self-responsibility. Review these from time to time.

Physical
- Loss of appetite
- Insomnia
- Frequent headaches
- Training fatigue that extends beyond 24 hours
- Pain or tenderness in joints
- Weight loss unassociated with caloric cutbacks
- Progressively deteriorating workouts
- A waking pulse rate which is 4 bpm higher than normal

Mental
- Feeling of depression unrelated to some major crisis
- Poor concentration and loss of alertness
- Waning interest in the opposite sex
- Frequent irritability and disatisfaction
- Lethargic feeling-loss of enthusiasm (Boredom)

Develop body wisdom—Know when your tail is wagging. This simply means getting in touch with yourself. My recommendations are based on scientific principles; still, you should not become a slave to these rules. On certain days you will really have a lot of zip. On other days you'll have a lot of zap. Don't push it. Or, do push it as your body tells you. Let your enthusiasm be your guide, which is why the last point listed above is perhaps the best guideline of all. When Pro, my hunting dog, quits wagging his tail late in the day, I know he's been hunted enough; his enthusiasm is gone. So, pretend you have a tail. As long as you feel like wagging it, all is okay. When you feel like it's dragging, cut back. With rest comes zest.

Defeating Boredom

High sensation seekers, be sure you vary your workout, workout environment, and other factors as much as possible to avoid the boredom you can't stand. You would do well to include several endurance activities to avoid monotony, keep your interest high, and reduce the likelihood of injuries. As an example, roller skating, cross-country skiing, or climbing are all good substitutes for running. Triathlons and orienteering are good events for you. Orienteering is a combination of running, hiking, map reading, and wanderlust. It's not crowded with people bearing down on you. You're close to nature with its kaleidoscope of colors mixed in with the challenge of the woods, infinite variety of terrain, and call of the wild. It offers relief from boredom at low expense. For more information, contact the U.S. Orienteering Federation, P.O. Box 1039, Ballwin, MO 63011.

One more thing; try adding some *music* to your workouts. Research (including my own) has shown that more work can be performed with less effort while listening to music. A seven-ounce portable radio might turn a workout into a concert (but not in high-traffic areas!). Ohio State Researcher Eric Miller found that runners conserved energy while running on a treadmill when listening to their portable. Try it with different sports and with different flavors of music. Experiment with different tempos. My own research found that subjects could run faster if the tempo of the music was slightly faster than their normal running cadence. Don't discount this aid as a motivational tool.

Those are your signposts. You have the roadmap because only *you* know how far you want to go. It's a question of self-fulfillment. Some of us have higher needs than others. The important thing is to try. The goal is *not* to be first across the finish line, or even overcoming boredom; the real goal is self-discovery.

CHAPTER 13
Selected References

Frederick, E.C. "Bone Jolt," *American Health*. July—August 1982.
Mirkin, Gabe. *The Sportsmedicine Book*. Little, Brown & Company, 1978.

CHAPTER 14
Happiness: The Ultimate Risk

Don't be afraid to risk being seen as crazy. In today's world, it is only your insanity that will keep you sane.
—Dr. Leo Buscaglia, Psychologist, author, noted speaker

Going Back in Time

If it were possible for you to enter a time machine and go back 40,000 years ago, to converse with your Cro-Magnon ancestors and pose the question, "Are you happy?", you might be rather surprised at the answer. You'd probably find that they had their ups and downs just like you do, that they had their share of good days and bad. Still, some distinctive differences would become apparent to you should you decide to stick around for a few days.

First you'd find that, because of the day to day rigors of survival, they didn't have leisure time, as you do, to sit around and think about their condition. Although they had celebrations and days of mourning, they weren't the philosopher you are. As our comforts and necessities become guaranteed we gain more time to sit around and pose the question "Why?" Cro-Magnon man, even though he had the same capacity for intelligence we do, did not have the sophisticated knowledge we gain from being born in the twentieth century. To put it bluntly, he didn't know what he was missing. His requirements for "happiness" were much simpler.

Second, after following the tribe around for a few days (assuming you could hold up) you would soon discover how busy they kept, for they were extremely active and very goal oriented—always seeking to improve the state of things such as the quality of tools, their hunting ploys, and other survival devices. Happiness for them probably meant being in harmony with nature, being able to gain a measure of control over its unpredictable events. To the extent that they were able to do so, they became more "sociable."

The Present Situation

But today we are the crowded masses. This means class distinctions, it means less available space to explore, and it means that social comparison is a fact of life. Your nearest neighbor is no longer geographically removed. From his close proximity he knows what kind of car you drive, what kind of clothes you wear, who your friends are, and whether the Zoysia grass you so painstakingly cultivated last spring has sprouted weeds to mar its aristocratic appearance. Happiness today is increasingly predicated upon being recognized as important to offset the feeling of being one among the masses, for each of us seeks (and needs) a sense of identity. But the simple tribe is now a "Supertribe", and the hierarchical order is not easily distinguished. So this can mean exhibiting all the entrapments of ease and comfort in an effort to communicate status. And with this struggle comes the negative risks of unhappiness and the distress that results.

Becoming Self-Actualized

One important lesson we can learn from our noble ancestors is to be *goal oriented*. Seek to improve ourselves, not in acquisition of things but in acquisition of knowledge. To early man and to primitive peoples of today, knowledge means survival. From early on the young are schooled in the tribal customs, beliefs, and folklore unique to a particular tribe. Usually through the fabric of religion the spiritual, physical, emotional, and social aspects of their being were integrated into a whole. It was important that all shared a fairly common belief system, or philosophy as we call it, to give life a sense of meaning. As colorful and full of childlike fancy and images of wrathful deities as such beliefs were, they still gave tribe members a sense of identity.

We also should build a knowledge system of beliefs that helps us make sense of the world. This is best accomplished not through a fragmented accumulation of facts but by building our own philosophies. Many great philosophies contain three elements; *Survival*—how to meet one's most basic needs and live as long and well as possible—*Growth* toward greater self-reliance (all cults promote a growth toward greater dependence), and *Spiritual Awareness,* that is, feeling, expressing, and sharing with others. The latter is what Erich Fromm called the "art of loving." All three require risk taking.

The famed psychologist Dr. Abraham Maslow studied peak performers to find out what motivated them. As a result, he developed a philosophy that unifies much of human behavior along a continuum from primitive survival instincts to the heights of spiritual experience. This need hierarchy, as he called it, does help us understand much of human motivation.

Maslow assumes you start life at the lowest level of the motivational

Maslow's Hierarchy

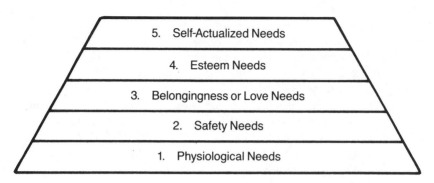

hierarchy, that is, he believes you are born with innate reflexes that help you satisfy your basic biological needs. Once you're blessed with biological life, however, you must secure some control over your physical environment. Thus, almost immediately after birth you begin to move up to the second level of the motivational hierarchy, that of safety needs. Once your basic physical wants (food, water, etc.) are secured, you will want to explore your physical environment. This exploration is necessary to reduce uncertainty about what the world has to offer, so you know what to expect from the world.

The next two rungs of the ladder involve the social environment. You need people to love, and you need people to love you. Part of these needs are satisfied by your family, but there are also work groups and various social organizations you can join. Not only can these groups offer you rewards for performing well, but they can help you learn what self-respect is all about. Through them you can better define your goals in life. As you achieve such goals your self-esteem improves. Maslow felt "esteem needs" were as important to human life as food and water.

If you're fortunate, you will finally reach the top rung of Maslow's hierarchy and achieve self-actualization, which means reaching your own greatest potential, doing the things you do best in your own unique way, and making your own unique contribution to society. It doesn't end here. Being self-actualized also means you feel a strong urge to help others get where you are, you sense a need to teach others the lessons you learned as you moved up the motivational hierarchy. This arises out of a love for all mankind and a desire to advance the human race as a whole.

Thus, whereas many psychologists reduce human behavior to a simple stimulus-response mechanism, Maslow's concept was quite holistic. It also allowed for free choice in determination of behavior, and this is why it fits in well with the positive risk-taking philosophies of this book. We can, by the kinds of risks we take, determine the quality of life. True, many things are influenced by our biological and social environments but we're still able to choose voluntarily, to weigh the risks and select the behaviors that best promote survival.

In reality, most of us fluctuate up and down the need hierarchy scale at different times or places in our life, yet still making choices, for better or worse. This brings us to what is an essential need and what isn't. Food is an essential need, no doubt. Is having a car a need? Okay. Is having a big luxury car a need? Is a $150,000 house a need when a $75,000 house will suffice? It seems obvious that needs beget needs. Once we "need" the $150,000 house, then we "need" to fill all those empty rooms, and the beat goes on, the never-ending theme of need. The more time we devote to all these needs, the less time we devote to becoming self-actualized.

Can primitive people be self-actualized? I believe they can, within the narrow cultural limits of their own societies. We hear of the Tonga Tribe in the South Pacific, whose people sacrificed a finger as a bloody sacrifice to placate the gods, and we think they were barbaric. Yet that was the norm. They would perhaps think we are barbaric in our attempts to hoard wealth, or maul someone to the ground in order to separate him from a small cylindrical object we call a football. We might also find it humorous that in some primitive societies, it is not the accumulation of wealth that bestows status, but rather the giving it away to others less fortunate.

> Prestige and leadership go to hunters who have food to dispense, hides to bestow, arrows to give, and horses to lavish upon favored friends, wayfaring visitors, and indigent neighbors. Management of wealth rather than its possession gives social recognition among primitive peoples. Social compulsion stimulates altruism, philanthropy, and good works. In civilization it has been easier to negate this principle than is the case in the primitive world, and the contrasts in wealth and poverty that occur within civilized societies are shocking to savages.

Wealth does not bestow self-actualization. It comes from the gaining of knowledge, development of one's potential, and the desire to help others do the same. Indeed, many of us may be less self-actualized than the savage we scorn.

The Risks of Being Yourself

In discussing happiness in greater detail, I should, once again, like to refer back to my own life; that is, my own motives for pursuing the risky feats described in Section I, I was living a respectful existence at the fourth rung of Maslow's hierarchy. I had everything we, in our materialistic society, deem worthwhile; a nice home, new sports car, closets full of suits and other nice clothes, and I was making a comfortable salary. All my basic needs were being met, but still I wasn't contented. I didn't feel my full talents were being used. I wanted more, wanted to explore some new realms of knowledge. I wanted to write about these experiences, and do more research on boredom and sensation-seeking behavior. As I did, I discovered a lot about myself: that I had an inordinately high need for physical challenges, and enjoyed researching the various risks each one presented and reducing the risks as much as possible. Admittedly, I'm different, crazy, weird, or whatever other adjectives we use to describe people who finally get fed up trying to be sane, sensible, and normal. But, I sure had a lot of fun. Better to have fun with your sanity suspect, than to be respectably bored.

Now, let's look at some of the risks you may face in order to be yourself (and happy).

> Being yourself may incur the wrath, criticism, or loss of love from others.
> Being yourself may result in a drastic change. This may be a divorce, change in jobs, etc.
> Being yourself may result in a reassessment of your whole value system, a whole reshuffling of priorities in order to find new meaning in life.

Thank God I chose my friends wisely and I had very loving and supportive parents. They all stood by me and were always there if I needed them. But, this isn't always the case, as the following case history demonstrates.

John was a lawyer. He made a lot of money, and had status and most of the material things all of us wish for. But he wasn't happy. In fact, he was depressed a great deal of the time. He didn't enjoy his profession and often felt as though life had no real meaning. Actually, John had never really wanted to be a lawyer. He went into law to please his father. His real interest was music

One afternoon, during a routine physical, John discovered he had cancer. After several weeks of retests and other medical opinions, his doctor relayed the sad news. John had six months to live. Thinking his life was nearly over, John gave up his law practice to pursue his musical interests. A strange thing began to happen; his cancer went into remission. Three years later, John is still going strong, he is truly happy, enjoying his life and his music to the fullest.

This is not an isolated case history. Dr. Lawrence LeShan, author of *You Can Fight For Your Life* has found that one of the key factors in the emotional life history of the cancer patient has been the suppression of his own devices.

> Frequently, I found, the cancer patient's own devices and wishes had been so completely repressed, and the self-alienation was so total that when at the start of therapy I asked the question, "What do YOU really want out of life?, the response would be a blank, astonished stare. That question had never been seen as valid.

Dr. LeShan, in one study found this sense of despair in 93 percent of cancer patients studied—yet it was found in only 3.5 percent of a control group (that had no cancer).

The case history of John, the lawyer, is an example of how being himself resulted in a drastic life change. In John's case it was precipitated by a life crisis. Why wait for a death sentence? Why not take the risk now? Remember, it's a positive risk because it leads to a genuine feeling of happiness, of being your real self. It may mean giving up a job or one kind of lifestyle for another. This may not (probably won't) be an easy thing to do. Happiness isn't always easy to achieve. You may have to give up income, status, and other security blankets in order to explore the real you. Another case history comes to mind.

At the age of twenty-seven, Brent had a master's degree in psychology and had been a counselor for the state vocational rehabilitation program for some two years. He did not enjoy this kind of work, even though he was making $18,000 per year. He was miserable. His discontentment flowed over into his home life, creating a sense of uneasiness and remoteness from his wife.

Brent had always been very artistic, and had developed hobbies in photography, art, and graphic layout. He thought he'd like to try advertising. Taking a positive risk, he took a job as marketing representative for an advertising agency in another city. His salary was $5,000 per year less and he had a 120-mile round trip to drive each day. He was able to obtain this position on the strength of freelance work he had done in graphic art production. Brent wasn't overjoyed with this new position but was relatively happy because he was learning a lot about marketing and advertising sales. A marketing package he put together earned him an award of excellence in a regional show. By the end of six months he was able to move to a much nicer (though demanding) job in Colorado, taking his wife with him. After two years, Brent finally found his "dream job": Director of Public Relations and Advertising for a Colorado resort that is one of the most luxurious hotels in the United States. His present salary is nearly double what he earned as a vocational counselor. Brent has taken a lot of risks in order to be himself, but now he's much happier.

Brent did a lot of risk taking in order to achieve happiness. He was able to get out of that rut so many people get into but are afraid to get out of. Being yourself isn't easy. It also means risking in other ways, by opening up your true feelings to others, whether expressing love, constructive criticism, or even anger. It means being totally honest in terms of what you can realistically expect of yourself and others. It also means self-responsibility, the ability to say, "If I'm not very happy, it's my own fault, and there are steps I can take to improve it."

Let's look again at some characteristics of the cancer-prone personality. Cancer is our second most prevalent disease.

Time and time again, in the test protocols, the short interviews, and the intensive psychotherapy sessions, it was clear that the cancer patients had difficulty in showing anger or aggression is defense of themselves. Other people would say, "She's a saint, or he's such a good, sweet man.

This attitude on the part of cancer patients studied in a clinic was related to their low self-esteem and inability to express their emotions. Dr. David Kissen, in his study of over 300 patients at a chest clinic, found one distinct personality characteristic that differentiated the cancer group from a control group: those with "a poor outlet for emotional discharge" were four and a half times more likely to have cancer. Dr. LeShan's findings were similar. Any situation that tended to disrupt the formation of strong, meaningful relationships increases the likelihood of cancer, based on mortality rates from Dr. LeShan's data.

By having the courage to express your feelings, good, bad, or otherwise, by having the courage to honestly communicate feelings of concern and love, you may thus be reducing your chances of getting cancer. Yes, it's a risk. You become vulnerable; you open up the possibility of rejection. But unless you do, you'll go on feeling "bottled up" and, as I've shown, this may be the greater risk. The payoff for expressing your feelings may be the best, most fulfilling relationship you've ever known.

Why People Won't Risk for Happiness

If exploring your own uniqueness is a necessary prerequisite for happiness, why don't more people take this risk? Why do they just go on day after day NOT being themselves? Dr. LeShan's work offers some insight:

They feel they can be themselves—and therefore unloved and alone—or, that they can get rid of themselves to be someone else and thus be loved.

In other words, they see it as a conflict between their "individuality" and their "popularity." In his book, *The Risks and Payoffs of Being Alive,* Dr. Peter Grant identifies four conditions needed for happiness—the "four A's"—attention, acceptance, approval, and affection. He portrays the self as a central "core" protected by five layers of armor, as in the illustration on page 196.

The outer layers are superficial and easily perceived by others. The inner layers are private, spiritual, and tough to penetrate. I'll briefly describe these layers.

Role Playing Most of us spend a great deal of our time role playing or pretending, since we are more concerned with how others see us than with nurturing our true selves.

Anxiety In this layer we occasionally take some risks in an attempt to be more genuine and honest but encounter some pain, sadness, and

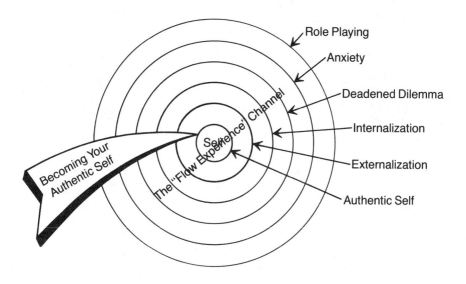

despair. The anxiety layer contains all the objections to being what we are.

Deadened Dilemma   Once we penetrate the anxiety layer, we feel we are not alive. We feel like a nothing. We're emotionally constipated. All our psychic energy is spent on maintaining the "living death" devoid of energy and enthusiasm.

Internalization   Our "life juice" resides here but these potential sources of energy and aliveness are frozen. We are aware of this aliveness but are still immobile and unable to explode into life at its fullest.

Externalization   We begin to turn our feelings outward. We become authentic; we're pulling the cork out. We can openly express many emotions.

Authentic Self   We become self-sufficient; we focus on the here and now and we become able to experience all kinds of deep feeling experiences. There is no need to manipulate others for emotional support.

Dr. Grant then goes on to systematically show how you can reach your authentic self in a way that reduces your risk of losing the *"four A's."* His whole approach is getting to know yourself, what you are, and where you are.

But let's go back for a moment to that authentic self, being able to enjoy the here and now, to fully experience the present and to be working toward self-actualization. Does this mean we won't find happiness until we've achieved our goal—a college degree, the right job, the right mate, the proper income, the style of living we've set for ourselves? The answer is no. Both factors can exist simultaneously. One needs to learn patience, to trust God, and sow the seeds that will eventually sprout. One must have a worthwhile plan, but recognize that all great plans are vintage wine. Have faith in yourself and in a higher spiritual energy, and develop a philosophy to guide your actions. Positive Risk Taking is one philosophy, Dr. Denis Waitley's *Ten Seeds of Greatness* (Revell Publish.) is another sound philosophy. The Christian philosophies of Dr. Robert Schuller are also a solid philosophy. Mine was meant to incorporate many aspects of wellness, though all have their own merits. They are all goal oriented and warn against expecting instant results. How often do we hear someone say, "If only I were able to have _____I could really be happy. I'll be happy just as soon as I _____. Once I finish _____I'm really gonna be happy." Happiness is made conditional, contingent upon reaching a specified end point. Certainly we need goals. We *should* aspire to some better self on down the road. But we can be happy NOW! As long as we have the knowledge we are headed in the right direction and that we are doing the best we can now, we deserve to feel happy. Far too many of us are swayed by social stresses and false gods. We believe that happiness is an "end-of-the-rainbow" event that will completely absorb us once we've reached a certain point, achieved a certain milestone, have a certain person, or are able to afford a certain item. This is *absolutely false!* Actually, happiness will never be achieved if we continue to think like this, for once we have obtained our desire it will not be long before we are again in search of something remote that promises self-fulfillment and happiness.

Happiness isn't the end of the rainbow, it IS the rainbow, a prism of never-ending colors, the trip as well as the arriving. We need to refocus. our values away from having to that of being. Let's look at another case history.

Fred, 48, owns an office supply company. He began as a salesman twenty years ago and gradually took over the whole company himself. He is about twenty-five pounds overweight, smokes, and consumes a lot of coffee to drive himself. Always in a hurry, always too impatient to really get to know anyone well except those who serve his business needs, he is locked in an incessant struggle with the clock. He tries to do more and more in less and less time. He can dictate a letter to his office over the car phone while devouring a Speedy Burger and planning new ways to cut costs. He moves in a very fast, jerky fashion, talks in rapid, hurried speech, and even attempts to hurry others' conversation by frequent interruptions and finishing their sentences. A total perfectionist in every sense, he always arrives 5 minutes early expecting the same of others.

He's extremely competitive about the smallest thing, even activities with his children. He rarely has time to attend cultural events with his wife, yet he thinks he is a good husband because he provides all the conveniences of life. He has no close friends and likes to brag about how many major accounts he has, how big his house is, and to compare his gross earnings with the next guy. Fred expends so much energy in his attempt to do more and more in less and less time that he needs a few Martinis to unwind at night.

According to Dr. Ray Rosemann and Dr. Meyer Friedman, authors of *Type A Behavior Pattern and Your Heart,* Fred's chances of having a heart attack in the next ten years are almost 100 percent. He is "Type A" in every way. He suffers from "hurry sickness," an emphasis on quantity rather than quality. Such a person will never be happy because he's always trying to outrun his shadow, unable to enjoy the here and now. He exemplifies the negative risk taker in many ways.

The sadness of it all, as Rosemann and Friedman point out, is that somewhere in the development of people like this, subtle messages were being communicated by society or parents (or both) that they'd be worthy of love, admiration, and respect only if they met a certain standard of excellence. This standard was perceived not in terms of *quality* of performance, that is how well, but rather *quantity* of performance or *how much.* The evidence that such continued striving leads to coronary heart disease is now very well established. In one study by these researchers, men in Type A category had seven times more heart disease than Type B men (categorized as slow, easy going, relaxed, yet with a purposeful attitude) even when diet and exercise habits were similar. To fill a life with deadlines to the exclusion of life's loveliness is a dreadful form of self-punishment. Such people will never find happiness as long as this syndrome continues.

Tips on Re-Engineering Your Life: Slowing Down

Here are some tips that could save your life and let you experience happiness if you exhibit Type A behavior patterns.

Revise your usual daily schedule of activities so as to eliminate as many events and activities as possible that do not directly contribute to your social economic well-being. Allow 5-10 minute rest breaks every hour or two.

Try to work in a place that promotes peace. Try to keep an orderly, neat work environment. Organize material into three categories. Those which need immediate attention, those requiring a delayed response, and those requiring no reply. Learn to delegate responsibility.

Consider your words. Learn to listen more. Learn to dismiss those who waste your time talking and avoid them. Try not to repeat yourself. Try to economize in good use of language.

At noon, try to escape and find a quiet place to gather your thoughts or just browse around with no one purpose in mind.

Forget five o'clock frenzy. Relax, realize you can finish up tomorrow or stay if necessary but don't find extra work beyond the necessary tasks.

Search for aloneness. Try to find your inner self. Go where there are no phones or interruptions. Perhaps even try flotation (Chapter 8).

Be brave enough to not get caught up in society's implied message of having rather than being. One good way to do this is to be aware of your spiritual and emotional needs and feed them daily. Invest in your friends welfare and find creative hobbies which you enjoy for their own sake. Remember, you cannot take things with you. Only your soul can move on.

Most Type A's are men. The female version is the "Type E," the everything woman, trying to make straight A's in all areas of her life. These women respond to demands from multiple areas. As Marjorie Shavitz writes in, *The Superwoman Syndrome:*

> Women, no matter how far they've gone in the career world don't think they're a success if they haven't succeeded in their personal lives.

Such women are also more susceptible to colds and flu as a result. Several suggestions; set meaningful priorities, learn to say "no" (chapter 11), exercise regularly, and relax your expectations. You can't be all things to everyone.

The Role of Play in Wellness

We saw how Type A behavior can interfere with the attainment of happiness. How can wellness help? A study at Duke University found that after ten weeks of walking and jogging, the number of Type A characteristics in subjects were reduced. In a similar study at Stanford Medical Center it was found that eight miles of jogging per week resulted in conversion from Type A behavior to Type B behavior. This change was not found in subjects who jogged less than eight miles per week. Type A behavior *can* be altered through fitness activities. Type A's need exercise to get them recentered. As we'll also see, it's a form of play.

It is also becoming well documented that exercise of the aerobic kind (endurance type) can effectively counter depression. Dr. Thaddeus Kostrubola, a psychiatrist from San Diego, is one of the leading advocates of running therapy and uses it on his patients with positive results. A number of scientific studies now show this change results from altering certain brain hormones.

Finally, as Dr. George Sheehan, a cardiologist, states:

> What our instincts tell us is that sports and athletics will show us how to satisfy the main urges of this generation: to possess one's experience rather

than be possessed by it, to live one's life rather than be lived by it . . . fitness through sport is not a test but a therapy; not a trial but a reward; not a question but an answer. . . . Exercise that is not play accentuates rather than heals the split between mind and body. Heed the inner calling to your own play. Listen to the person you were and are and can be. Then do what you do best and feel best at, something you would do for nothing, something that gives you security and self-acceptance and a feeling of completion; even moments when you are fused with your universe and your creator . . . there is no better test for play than the desire to be doing it when you die.

Dr. Mihaly Csikszentmihalyi, a psychology professor at the University of Chicago and author of *Beyond Boredom and Anxiety—The Experience of Play in Work and Games,* has conducted extensive research into intrinsic motivation, that is, trying to resolve the question as to why people do something for nothing, when there doesn't appear to be any tangible reward, such as money, as a form of motivation. He labels such activities *autotelic activities.* He writes,

It is important to find out why people engage in autotelic activities because a community that knows how to create autotelic personalities will be more happy and more efficient than one which relies only on external motivation.

The primary reason, he finds, why people will do something purely for its own sake is to achieve a "flow experience." During flow they become so focused upon what they are doing, they merge or become one with the activity. Time collapses, there is no past, there is no future, only the beautiful *now.* A person in flow experiences a loss of ego awareness because what they are doing is so enjoyable they become unaware of anything else in the environment besides the actual demands of the activity itself. The activity, as Dr. Csikszentmihalyi discovered, can be rock climbing, dancing, chess, surgery, or any activity in which there is total involvement of mind and body. High-intensity sports seem to provide the best opportunities. The primary ingredients are total concentration, a feeling of control over the demands of the activity or environment, a focusing of attention within a very narrow stimulus field, and a desire to perform the activity for the experience itself rather than the end result. People in flow temporarily forget their identity and its problems. The satisfaction of oneness, heightened perception, and control supercedes all else. As some rock climbers put it,

You feel more alive; internal and external don't get confused. The task at hand is so rich in its complexity and pull that your intensity as a conscious subject is diminished; a more subtle loss of self than forgetfulness.

It's a pleasant feeling of total involvement. You become like a robot . . . no, more like an animal . . . getting lost in kinesthetic sensations . . . a panther powering up the rock

For the first time, we noticed tiny bugs that were all over the walls, so tiny that they were barely noticeable. While belaying I stared at one for fifteen full minutes, watching him move and admiring his brilliant red color. . . . How could one ever be bored with so many good things to see and feel! This unity with our joyous surroundings, this ultra-penetrating perception, gave us a feeling that we had not had for years.

What occurs is an intense seeing, the vision induced by physical exertion combined with an activity that requires a high degree of skill, the result being a transformation of material objects and the generalized "oceanic feeling of the supreme sufficiency of the present." Such profound experiences of flow are called *deep play,* although *micro-flow* experiences and the enjoyment they bring may be had often during a typical day if one pursues activities for their own sake rather than merely for material gain.

In today's society, people do not enjoy flow experiences as frequently as our ancestors probably did. There are two reasons for this change. First, there are many more distractions in our complex modern world, one is rarely able to focus on a limited stimulus field for very long.

Second, most employers don't understand how to structure jobs to make them more enjoyable and challenging. Games, sports, and various art forms have developed along such structural lines.

But work and education, two institutions that occupy most of our time are not built to provide optimal intrinsic motivation partly because of the ingrained cultural distinction between work and play, or study and play. People tend to suspect that if work is enjoyable it must not be productive.

Dr. Csikszentmihalyi's research has shown otherwise. Flow can promote happier workers and can be achieved more often if employees are allowed to feel a greater sense of control, to structure time rather than be structured by it. Corporate wellness programs that provide on-site fitness facilities are examples of how play can be integrated into the work environment. The recent trend of companies using "flex time" for their employees is also an excellent strategy for giving workers a feeling of more control over the demands and structure of their jobs.

As I've already implied, flow experiences require challenges, to create the activation and arousal necessary for flow to occur. I have offered you many challenges in this book, while always trying to give you the skills necessary to successfully meet those challenges. The more flow you can experience in your life, the more happiness you should experience.

Dr. Csikszentmihalyi has described a model that illustrates the relationship between these two variables, challenge and skill level. As the model illustrates, when the risk situation (the challenge: asserting yourself, running a marathon, or taking on some new demand at work) is greater than your skill level, anxiety will result. When your skill level is well

Model of the Flow State

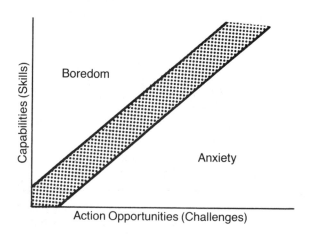

Action Opportunities (Challenges)

beyond the challenge (menial tasks), then boredom is very likely. Happiness then, means enhancing your flow opportunities.

When a person believes that his action opportunities are too demanding for his capabilities, the resulting stress is experienced as anxiety; when the ratio of capabilities is higher, but the challenges are still too demanding for his skills, the experience is worry. The state of flow is felt when the opportunities for action are in balance with the person's skills; the experience is then autotelic. When skills are greater than opportunities for using them, the state of boredom results; this state again fades into anxiety when the ratio becomes too large.

The writing of this book provided me with innumerable flow experiences, I could spend an entire day never knowing where the hours went. The building climb provided me with flow, once I felt my skills were in balance with the challenge.

What happens if we don't get enough flow experiences? Dr. Csikszentmilalyi found that when subjects were denied play and flow experiences, they reported feeling more fatigued, less relaxed, had more headaches, more negative attitudes, felt less creative, less able to concentrate, became less spontaneous, more irritable, depressed, and had the feeling of having been turned into a machine. As this researcher summed it all up;

> To be able to do things that may not appear necessary to a person's survival gives one a feeling of effectance, of being in control of one's actions rather than a pawn in the hands of determinate fate. In addition, this kind of behavior probably regulates the amount of stimulation available to the organism, by supplying novelty in a barren environment or reducing input when the stim-

ulation is excessive. Obviously, when such behavior is not available to people, for whatever reason, the attention process is disrupted, the control of stimulus input breaks down, and serious consequences (acute psychotic breakdown) may result. At the very least, people deprived even for a short time show significant negative effects.

Don't take life too seriously; you may be harming your immune system, as an exciting new field of *psycho-immunology* shows.

Happiness, Wellness, and Psycho-Immunology

The immune system is our vigilant sentinel that encounters foreign substances (bacteria, viruses, dust, or pollen), and then destroys them or renders them harmless. A number of studies are now providing strong evidence that psychological factors can increase or decrease the competence of this system. For example, one Australian researcher found that the death of a husband or wife can lessen the grieving spouse's immunological competence.

At John Hopkins University, Dr. Caroline Thomas correlated psychological factors with the long-term health records of 1,337 medical students between 1948 and 1964. One of the strongest predictors of cancer, mental illness, and suicide, she discovered, was "lack of closeness to parents," and a negative attitude toward one's family.

Epidemiologist Leonard Syme of Berkeley, California, after adjusting for risk factors such as smoking and medical history, still concluded that those people who had few close contacts with others were dying at a rate of two to three times those who had close friends they could turn to.

Another study found that mice injected with cancer cells and then put in isolation developed tumors much more frequently than those who were maintained with their cage mates.

What this means is that as we become happy, we sort of self-immunize ourselves against potential disease and illness. The reverse is probably true. As we become more unhappy, despondent, and hopeless, our natural immunity decreases, leaving us more vulnerable to diseases like cancer.

New research has finally uncovered what may well be the "missing link" explaining why negative emotions and attitudes cause illness or disease. Receptor sites (specialized areas for transmission of nerve impulses) have been discovered on the surface of white blood cells. The white blood cells are part of our immune system. What this means is that a relay system has finally been discovered linking the nervous system to the immune response itself. Dr. Robert Ader of the University of Rochester School of Medicine and Marvin Stein at City College of New York are two of the leading pioneers in this new field of study.

No matter how many times you have failed in the past, you must continue to try new behaviors. This is positive risk taking. Otherwise, you will become a victim of *learned helplessness*. An example from research will explain this concept. Wild rats, forced to swim until exhaustion, lasted sixty hours before they drowned. Rats that were held firmly in the researcher's hand so that they could not escape, were only able to swim for thirty minutes before drowning. The handled rats acted as if they were helpless. If, however, the rats were allowed to wriggle free from the experimenter's grip, so that they believed they escaped (a success), this helplessness did not occur, and they could swim for an extended period of time. A similar version of this experiment has been conducted with humans, using shock as a form of punishment from which they could not escape. Dr. Richard Carney, author of *Risk Taking Behavior,* states that good risk takers are able to change their strategy, moving in a more conservative or more liberal direction, as necessary, until they succeed. The message is *keep trying;* don't be afraid to experiment.

Wellness, with its emphasis on peak performance (self-actualization), rather than normal levels, can be assisted in two key ways. One is through laughter and the other is through touch, specifically, hugging. To do *both* of these things on a regular basis will not only make you a more happy, loving person, but also help immunize you against disease. Let me explain why.

Hugging seems to be a miracle medicine that can resolve many physical and emotional problems facing all Americans, experts say. Researchers have discovered that hugging can help you live longer, protect you against illness, cure depression, strengthen family relationships, and even cure insomnia. By lifting depression, it tunes up the body's immune system.

Researchers have discovered that when a person is touched for at least 15 minutes the amount of hemoglobin in the blood increases significantly. Hemoglobin carries vital supplies of oxygen in the blood to all organs of the body, including the heart and brain. An increase in hemoglobin tones up the whole body and speeds recovery from illness. The warm and meaningful embrace can have a very positive effect on people, especially during periods of excessive stress and tension. One psychiatrist found that painful headaches, backaches, and stomach aches in married couples responded to greater intimacy. The couples, once they openly expressed their feelings and began to touch each other, had relief of their pain, even when it hadn't responded to traditional drug therapy. It was certainly a factor in my own life during some of the fears I had to confront. A prescription of four good hugs per day from family or friends should help keep you well.

Laughter also is wellness medicine. Norman Cousins, in his *Anatomy Of An Illness,* described how watching tapes of *Candid Camera* TV shows provoked positive emotions of joy and happiness because of the laughter they created. This, he feels, played a major role in helping defeat the "incurable" disease he was suffering from. De Kalb General Hospital in Atlanta, Georgia, and Shawnee Mission Medical Center in Kansas City have already designated laughter rooms to provide therapy for cancer patients. Lively music as well as videotapes of Laurel and Hardy films and *Candid Camera* shows are used to promote laughter in those rooms. A prescription of ten laughs per day should keep you well.

Both hugging and laughing involve risk taking, especially if you haven't been doing them already because you risk being seen as different or out of place. They're both positive risks with a high wellness payoff.

As I close this chapter, I should like to leave you with one of my favorite poems. In a sense, the author is protesting the false facade of success. The individual portrayed has taken the greatest risk of all, not really living his own life. There is a lesson here for all of us.

Richard Cory

Whenever Richard Cory went down town,
We people on the pavement looked at him:
He was a gentleman from sole to crown,
Clean favored, and imperially slim.

And he was always quietly arrayed,
And he was always human when he talked;
But still he fluttered pulses when he said,
"Good Morning," and he glittered when he walked.

And he was rich—yes, richer than a king—
And admirably schooled in every grace:
In short, we thought that he was everything
To make us wish that we were in his place.

So on we worked, and waited for the light,
And went without the meat, and cursed the bread;
And Richard Cory, one calm summer night
Went home and put a bullet through his head.

—Edwin Arlington Robinson

CHAPTER 14
Selected References

Booth, Gotthard. *Psychobiological Aspects of Spontaneous Regressions of Cancer,* Chapter 11 from Stress and Survival, (ed.) Charles A. Garfield, C.V. Mosby Company, 1979.

Csikszentmihalyi, Mihaly. *Beyond Boredom and Anxiety—The Experience of Play in Work and Games.* Jossey-Bass, 1975.

LeShan, Lawrence. *You Can Fight for your Life—Emotional Factors in the Causation of Cancer.* M. Evans Company, 1977.

Locke, Steven E. "Mind and Immunity: An Annotated Bibliography 1976–82." *Institute for the Advancement of Health,* 16 East 53rd, New York, NY 10022.

Pelletier, Kenneth. "The Missing Link—How Emotions Influence Disease." *Medical Self-Care,* Fall 1984.

The Future: Wellness or Self-Destruction?

Nations have passed away and left no traces, and history gives the naked cause of it. One single, simple reason in all cases, they fell because their people were not fit.

—Rudyard Kipling

Summary

1. I have tried to show you that to be a good risk taker, you must apply the wellness concepts (good nutrition, fitness, stress control, etc.) to succeed in the great enterprise of life.

2. By having some knowledge, however scant, of our primitive ancestors and how rapid the changes of this century have been, we can gain a better perspective upon ourselves. This is especially true regarding our biological needs for stimulation which, as I have indicated, can result in behaviors injurious to your health. Rapid change of any kind requires new behaviors, in this case, learning to take the right kinds of risks.

3. In order to get the most from life, you should take the offensive, take charge, so to speak, of your own destiny. Living life on the defense, that is, sidestepping or merely trying to parry the blows thrown at you by people or situations will in the long run only cause excessive strain and unhappiness.

4. Whereas a certain degree of unpredictability is a natural consequence of life, we ALL can control (to a very large degree) those factors which affect our own health and stability. By doing so, we increase the odds of achieving our goals and enjoying the satisfactions thereof.

5. Modern society, while offering us opportunities never before dreamed possible, also has its excesses, and we can easily become a victim, rather than a master, of our technological advances. Self-control was an essential issue, enjoy the modern world by controlling it rather than vice versa.

6. Generally speaking, health and human values go hand in hand. As the body or mind becomes polluted, there will be a shift from greater spiritual growth toward moral decline and decay, the emphasis on *having* rather than *being*.

7. Finally, I have tried to motivate you, to show you the vast possibilities of the human spirit that can be achieved through wellness skills like visualization, open communication, and the pursuit of those qualities and behaviors that make each of us unique. To emphasize some of the concepts in the book I described my own odyssey as a risk taker, and proposed the heroic goal as an antidote to boredom and mediocrity.

The Future

Where are we going? Will we follow the same pattern of the once-great civilizations like Rome and Greece that fell into decline because of internal decay? The signs are there.

Crime is at an all-time high. The United States ranks near the top in the number of suicides and homicides per 100,000 adult population compared to other countries. And when it comes to the number of alcoholics (with or without complications), we top the list of other countries. The incidence of alcoholism is a symptom of mental and emotional instability.

A study released by the National Institutes of Mental Health on more than 9,500 people found that 20 percent of Americans suffer from some form of mental illness in any given six-month period. Such illnesses include depression, anxiety, schizophrenia, phobias, drug addiction, and a variety of other disorders. We entertain an erroneous notion in this country that when the frequency of some disorder becomes so widespread that it is fairly common, then the disorder itself must not be so bad and we make it an acceptable form of behavior. Homosexuality is one example. Considered a mental illness until 1973, it became ''normal'' when the American Psychological Association voted it out. Erich Fromm, world renowned psychiatrist and author of *The Sane Society* had some interesting comments in this regard:

> Many psychiatrists and psychologists refuse to entertain the idea that society as a whole may be lacking in sanity. They hold that the problem of mental health in a society is only that of the number (%) of ''unadjusted'' individuals, and not that of a possible maladjustment of the culture itself . . . the possibility of what I call ''Pathological Normalcy'' . . . the fact that millions of people share the same vices does not make these vices virtues. . . . Nothing could be further from the truth''.

The issues in question then are: What constitutes a ''normal'' person? What constitutes a happy person in optimal physical and mental health? How and under what conditions is this best achieved? Risk-taking concepts can provide the answer.

One cannot stop the world and get off. We cannot go back to the simplicity and originality of Jacques Rousseau's "noble savage"." There is no Arcadia or Golden Era to which we can return and live in bliss. To live is to struggle. A satisfying life is not one without ordeals, failures, and tragedies, but one where each of us challenges our own physical and social environment. But the environment must be managed so as to provide immense diversity to accommodate all the varieties of human expression. As Dr. Rene DuBois, author of *The Animal Human* writes:

> Technology should have as its most important goal the creation of environments in which the widest range of human potentialities can unfold. . . . Man has been highly successful as a biological species because he is adaptable. He can hunt or farm, be a meat eater or a vegetarian, live in the mountains or by the seashore, be a loner or a team member, function in a democratic society or totalitarian state. History shows, on the other hand, that societies which were efficient because they were highly specialized rapidly collapsed when conditions changed. A highly specialized society, like a narrow specialist, is rarely very adaptable.
>
> Cultural homogenization and social regimentation resulting from the creeping monotony of overorganized and overtechnicized life, of standard patterns of education, mass communication, and entertainment, will make it progressively more difficult to exploit fully the biological richness of civilization. We must shun uniformity of surroundings as much as absolute conformity in behavior and tastes. We must strive instead to create as many diversified environments as possible. Richness and diversity of physical and social environments constitute an essential criteria of functionalism, whether in the planning of cities, the design of dwellings, or the management of individual life.
>
> Diversity may result in some loss of efficiency. It will certainly increase the variety of challenges, but the more important goal is to provide the many kinds of soil that will permit the germination of seeds now dominant in man's nature. Man innovates and thus fully expresses his humanness by responding creatively, even though often painfully, to stimuli and challenges. Societies and social groups that have removed themselves into the pleasure garden, where all was designed for safety and comfort have achieved little else and have died in this snug world.

The wellness physician, Dr. Halbert Dunn, who first coined the term high-level wellness, said that diversity to thought, uniqueness of personality, and variety in self-expression were essential features of that term. They all involve risk taking.

The noted British historian Arnold Toynbee sees many parallels between the past and our current path in the western world. After making a study of some twenty-one major civilizations covering a 6,000-year period, he concluded that all great civilizations fell into decline because they became poor risk takers. All these great civilizations prospered because of risks taken to promote growth. Examples included active exploration of the environment (to allow for geographical expansion), creativity and inventiveness, and also social risks aimed at increasing the size and communication skills of its people. So what we see, in effect, are forces promoting growth and forces promoting decline, the struggle between positive risk taking and negative risk taking. Toynbee called this the struggle between the material and the spiritual forces of life. Indeed, he felt that greed was a universal characteristic of humans, and that in order for a civilization to survive, the spiritual forces must predominate and the material forces must be held in check.

The signs of decay are evident in all the negative risks or choices we take. As I have enumerated throughout this book, these include poor health habits, gluttony, greed, crime, declining moral values, various forms of escapism (drugs, cults, and not expressing our feelings). These are all forms of internal decay. Statistics show that the incidence of homicides has tripled since 1950, the incidence of suicides is up 10% since 1970, and divorce rates have more than doubled since 1965 and a Justice Department study found that youths born in 1958 are committing violent crimes at three times the rate as those born in 1945. These are all barometers which indicate that we are indeed entering a period of moral decadence as we approach the year 2000.

Will we succumb to this fate as a nation? The answer depends on you. There are winners in life, the positive risk takers, and there are losers in life, the negative risk takers. The choice is yours. Whatever your religion, I'm sure we all agree that life seems to be an ongoing struggle between the material and spiritual forces of life. If you believe as I do, in the goodness of all people, in free will, in man's freedom to respond with all his heart and soul to a problem, then you know that we owe it to ourselves and future generations to go on risking, in the wellness direction (wellness continuum, chapter 1). This is what separates us from the lower forms of life. We do not simply evolve from mutations, we evolve from conscious actions, actions and decisions directed toward our own welfare, and that of others.

As I close this book, I would remind you once more that wellness goes far beyond nutrition and fitness. These are only means to an end. The essence of wellness is high goal setting, finding challenges (and achieving them) to offset the boredom and poor health so commonplace in modern society. Thus, wellness is a spiritual reawakening, a calling forth to the spirit of man, to regain the enthusiasm of the child, and to heed the call of the trumpet. It is to know when your time is done, that you risked often and well, that you fulfilled the purpose for which you came, that you finished a winner in the game of life.

In the nineteenth century the problem was that *God is dead;* in the twentieth century the problem is that *man is dead.* In the nineteenth century inhumanity meant cruelty; in the twentieth century it means schizoid self-alienation. The danger of the past was that men became slaves. The danger of the future is that men may become robots. True enough, robots do not rebel. But, given man's nature, robots cannot live and remain sane, they become 'Golems' they will destroy their world and themselves because they cannot stand any longer the boredom of a meaningless life.

—Dr. Erich Fromm

CHAPTER 15
Selected References

DuBois, Rene. *So Human An Animal.* Charles Scribner's Sons.

Fromm, Eric. *The Sane Society.* Rinehart, 1955.

Toynbee, Arnold. *Civilization on Trial.* Oxford University Press, 1948

Index